Contents

D0541913

About the author

Maureen Boyle is a senior lecturer at Thames Valley University. She has been a midwife for more than 20 years, and currently continues her clinical practice at St Mary's Hospital in Paddington, London. She has published widely, most recently including *Emergencies Around Childbirth: A Handbook for Midwives* (2002, Radcliffe Publishing).

1

Introduction

Infection is the leading cause of death in the human population.[12]

Midwives will rarely have to care for a woman with a serious infection, and in most cases even the most extreme infection will respond to treatment and the outcome will be good. However, until the 1930s infection was the main cause of maternal death in the UK,[1] and despite excellent progress in the care of these women, during the period 2000–02 sepsis was still the fifth commonest cause of maternal mortality in the UK (and estimated to be the second commonest cause of maternal death worldwide).[2] Although the relatively small number of deaths among women in the UK can be seen as a success, it must be remembered that any infection may also lead to short- or long-term morbidity, which can influence or even permanently change a woman's life.

It is acknowledged that any infection in a pregnant woman may impact on the fetus and newborn, and indeed some postnatal maternal infections may also disadvantage the baby by potentially compromising breastfeeding and/or maternal–infant interactions. Although consideration of the baby is beyond the remit of this book, it must also be remembered that a woman can be cured herself, but may tragically lose her baby to intrauterine infection. The importance of this subject is beyond dispute.

This book will only consider the healing of maternal wounds and potential complications – infectious diseases such as HIV, TB or malaria, although potentially of growing concern for the midwife, are beyond the remit of this book. Similarly, emotional and/or psychological healing is too large a subject to be considered here. It is of course assumed that any adverse outcome of pregnancy will have psychological effects, some of which may be extreme. This topic is receiving deservedly increased attention, especially with the identification of post-traumatic stress syndrome associated with birth, and there are many recent publications on this subject.

Infection can complicate many normal procedures or situations, with sometimes fatal results. The most recent *Confidential Enquiries into Maternal Deaths in the UK*[2] reports women dying following routine amniocentesis, and also after a water birth and other uncomplicated deliveries.

The postnatal period is perhaps the most vulnerable period for healthy women – as this is the time when most women will neglect their own health while they prioritise care of the newborn. Many women will make efforts to optimise their health for conception, and some for the 'ordeal' of labour, but little has been written about preparing for the postnatal period when healing, establishing breastfeeding, sleep deprivation and perhaps limited nutrition make heavy demands on a woman's health. These are all issues where the advice and support of the midwife could potentially make a significant difference.

The immune system of most women can cope with the various assaults during pregnancy, childbirth and perhaps the puerperium, without succumbing to disease or infection. However, this will require resources, and the immune system will need to be activated to protect the woman from every breach of its defences – from a venepuncture or urinary catheter to an exposed placental site – so by the time the woman reaches the puerperium her resources may be depleted. At this stage the extra energy output necessary may be enough to make a previously healthy woman feel unhealthy, and even if she does not actually become ill, she may certainly not feel well, and the early days of motherhood may be compromised. Maternal functional health may be decreased for months after delivery, even in individuals with no complications. It has been shown that mothers can feel very unprepared for this, and want more information about their health.[3]

An overwhelming complaint during the puerperium is tiredness.[4] This may be due not only to interrupted sleep, but also to the body's need to rebuild its defences. Midwives need to be aware of how the immune system works at this time (*see* Chapter 2) and to ensure that women have the information necessary to maintain a healthy immune system.

Even if there are no complications at all, there are wounds that need to heal following childbirth, and Chapter 3 considers the theory of wound healing. Over the past 20–25 years wound healing has become a discipline in its own right,[5] and most midwives will have access to specialists in this field whom they can use as a resource if questions arise about how to treat a difficult wound or which dressing to use. However, the vast majority of women will not require specialist care, and the midwife should have an overview of how wounds heal in order to ensure that she can offer advice to enhance the wound-healing process.

Chapters 5 and 6 contain a more detailed discussion of the two wounds of childbirth over which the midwife has most influence, namely the perineal and Caesarean section wounds. These chapters include descriptions of the specific healing that takes place in these two areas, together with the potential complications and treatments. Chapter 5 also includes a list of possible midwifery actions that could 'protect' the perineum, as a reduction in trauma that would decrease the need for healing would be the best possible outcome.

Wounds and infections are not always a priority in midwifery care, although the midwife has a very strong influence over the woman's well-being in these areas. In the most recent *Confidential Enquiries into Maternal Deaths in the UK*,[2] 13 deaths were considered to be directly due to genital tract sepsis, and the assessors found some elements of suboptimal care in 80% of the cases considered. Of particular concern was the lack of appreciation of the possible speed of an infectious course. It is particularly important for midwives to note that of the five women who died after a vaginal delivery, four only became ill after discharge home from hospital.

Early discharge of a woman from hospital care will put the community midwife in the primary position for being alert to any serious infection and acting promptly. Indeed historically, when the role of the midwife was initially defined, the reason for postnatal visits was to prevent and/or treat infection.[6] Today, despite the increasing number of issues that the midwife must address in the community, it is worth remembering that for some women this will continue to be a vital part of the midwife's role.

Although it is obviously important for a midwife to be able to identify infection as soon as possible for the well-being of the woman concerned, she also has other responsibilities in this area. Morbidity around the time of childbirth has always been a very under-documented area, especially with regard to sepsis. Following the now routine early discharge from hospital, most infection is recognised by the community midwife, who will then refer the woman to her general practitioner (GP) for treatment. Statistics are rarely kept on particular infections or on procedures that may lead to infection, thus limiting the lessons that can be learned. It is the responsibility of the midwife to give feedback on infection in the community, and if they are in place, routine risk management procedures may be the most effective route for passing on this information.[7] Regular audit may identify areas that need improvement, and there is some evidence that where regular feedback mechanisms are in place, a decrease in infection may occur.[8]

Too often midwives can become complacent because they care for healthy young women with effective immune systems who can usually handle any assault. However, maintaining good practice at all times will ensure that the woman who is vulnerable does not suffer any ill effects from our care.

Women are more susceptible to some infections during pregnancy, but the commonest time for an infection to occur is during the postnatal period. When the wounds following childbirth need to heal, the efficiency of the immune system is dependent on many factors, ranging from genetic inheritance to how much sleep the woman had the previous night. Successful immune activation is the usual response to minor or even major assaults, but at what cost is this?

Fatigue is a symptom that most new mothers would recognise. In research studies tiredness has been demonstrated to last for more than six to seven months in some cases,[9] and although it has been shown to be associated with anaemia and entonox use in labour,[4] for many women it will be the care of a newborn and perhaps other children, together with the general anxiety that often accompanies the arrival of a new baby, that will cause interrupted sleep and therefore general fatigue. Sleep is vital for wound healing and the prevention of infection, and this is one of the reasons why a new mother may be susceptible to infection. She may also be too caught up in caring for the newborn to pay attention to her own nutrition. If she then encounters a challenge to her immune system, the exposure to pathogens will lead to an increase in metabolic activity as her body's defences mount a defence. In a vulnerable new mother who may also be physically challenged by the normal healing and body changes following childbirth, along with breastfeeding and psychological stress associated with care of the newborn, the immune system may simply be unable to cope.

Prevention of infection is the responsibility of all staff, but in particular those involved in direct care.[10] Although these days care on a postnatal ward may be undertaken by various categories of staff, the midwife is the individual with primary responsibility for the well-being of the new mother,[11] and it is therefore up to her to set standards and supervise others to ensure that they maintain best practice. It may also be necessary for all midwives to ensure that their own care of IV infusion sites, urinary catheters and other routine potential sources of infection is up to date. Chapter 9 reviews some of these aspects, to ensure that midwifery skills are of a standard which ensures that the woman is not put at unnecessary risk. In Chapter 8 some of the less common infections that may complicate wounds will be identified, such as methicillin-resistant *Staphylococcus aureus* (MRSA) and necrotising fasciitis, and these will be discussed along with some more common infections.

In present-day practice, women often look to midwives for advice about areas that have not traditionally been part of our care. Nutrition is one such subject, and it is such a vital part of health that it impacts on the success of all midwifery care. However, nutrition is a huge subject, so Chapter 4 will only contain an overview of the part that nutrition plays in wound healing.

Many women in the UK today are accessing complementary therapies, and indeed many midwives are also becoming knowledgeable about and even obtaining qualifications in these fields. This is another area of changing midwifery practice, and Chapter 7 will consider some of the commonest complementary therapies and their suggested roles in healing.

It is acknowledged that there are areas of overlap in this book, in particular between the chapters on the immune system and wound healing. This is inevitable because both of these systems serve to protect the body. Similarly, there are other areas of potential repetition due to the fact that systems are interlinked. For example, because the immune system is necessary for wound healing, nutrition is necessary for both, and some specific treatments and/or lifestyle issues can influence (positively or negatively) the uptake of nutrients and the working of the immune system, as well as being identified as risk factors for perineal or Caesarean section wound infection.

It is the aim of this book to include up-to-date, evidence-based information on wound healing that is relevant to midwifery care. However, a brief consideration of the history of infection and wounds in relation to childbirth may form an interesting foundation.

Historically, infection around the time of childbirth is not a new concept. Puerperal (or 'childbed') fever has been noted since ancient times, and Hippocrates provided clear descriptions of cases around 400 BC. In Britain as well as in the rest of Europe, the 1700s saw the beginning of 'lying-in' hospitals or wards as part of general hospitals. These were mostly for poor women, as those who were better off usually chose to have their babies at home. However, there were outbreaks of puerperal fever both in the community and in hospitals, and these outbreaks were usually severe.[12]

The fact that puerperal fever was spread from person to person (in particular by birth attendants) was only very slowly realised. Dr Alexander Gordon published work in Aberdeen in 1795 which demonstrated how the disease followed various midwives and doctors (including himself) from woman to woman. His 'theory' was not accepted, although other authors published similar findings, including Collins in Dublin in 1835, Holmes in the USA in 1843, Simpson in Edinburgh in 1850 and Semmelweiss in Vienna in 1861. However, as a result of a general movement towards cleanliness, reducing overcrowding, and preventing attendants from working on other general wards while providing care for patients in lying-in wards, hospital deaths from puerperal fever began to be controlled. For example, in Queen Charlotte's Hospital in London, the number of deaths fell from 26.8 per 1000 in 1875–79 to 4.5 per 1000 in 1900–02.[13]

However, in the 1900s puerperal fever became more common in the community, rather than in hospitals, as GPs and midwives were less likely to follow the antiseptic and aseptic practice that was now common in hospitals.

The next dramatic fall in the number of deaths from puerperal fever occurred following the introduction of prontosil (a sulphonamide) in the late 1930s. After 1945 penicillin also became available, which contributed to the continuing downward trend in deaths from puerperal fever.

Comparison of present-day outcomes with those of the fairly recent past could be described as a success story. Drug therapy and the adoption of aseptic procedures (as well as control and treatment of blood loss, and generally improved health and nutrition for women leading to reduced susceptibility) mean that severe infection is no longer a common complaint. However, although there are no longer epidemics of puerperal fever in the UK, wound infection still has the potential to cause long-term suffering and, less frequently, the tragedy of loss, both for individual women and for their families.

References

1   Drife J (2002) Lessons from the confidential enquiries in the UK. In: A MacLean and J Neilson (eds) *Maternal Morbidity and Mortality.* RCOG Press, London.

2   Lewis G (ed.) (2004) *Why Mothers Die: confidential enquiries into maternal deaths in the UK: 2000–2002.* RCOG Press, London.

3   Kline C, Martin D and Deyo R (1998) Health consequences of pregnancy and childbirth as perceived by women and clinicians. *Obstet Gynecol.* **92:** 842–8.

4   MacArthur C, Lewis M and Knox E (1991) *Health after Childbirth.* HMSO, London.

5   Baxter H (2002) How a discipline came of age: a history of wound care. *J Wound Care.* **11:** 383–92.

6   Abbott H, Bick D and McArthur C (1997) Health after birth. In: C Henderson and K Jones (eds) *Essential Midwifery.* Mosby, London.

7   Bates C (2002) Assessing and managing risk in midwifery practice. In: M Boyle (ed.) *Emergencies Around Childbirth: a handbook for midwives.* Radcliffe Medical Press, Oxford.

8   Brocklehurst P (2001) Infection and caesarean section. In: A MacLean, L Regan and D Carrington (eds) *Infection and Pregnancy.* RCOG Press, London.

9   Bick D, MacArthur C, Knowles H *et al.* (2002) *Postnatal Care: evidence and guidelines for management.* Churchill Livingstone, Edinburgh.

10 Ayliffe G, Fraise A, Geddes A *et al.* (2000) *Control of Hospital Infection: a practical handbook* (4e). Arnold, London.

11 Nursing and Midwifery Council (2004) *Midwives' Rules and Standards.* Nursing and Midwifery Council, London.

12 Ayliffe G and English M (2003) *Hospital Infection: from miasmas to MRSA.* Arnold, London.

13 Loudon I (2000) *The Tragedy of Childbed Fever.* Oxford University Press, Oxford.

2

The immune system and its response

The immune system is one of the most complex systems of the body, involving many cells and molecules, the actions of most of which are inter-related. These multiple activities are not confined to one area or organ, but can be found throughout the body. The basic function of the immune system is to maintain the internal environment of the body, which it achieves by:

- acting to remove cells that die naturally
- fighting infection
- contributing to wound healing.

During pregnancy there is evidence of both enhancement of and a reduction in the immunological response, probably caused by placental hormones and changes in corticosteroid levels. White blood cells (especially neutrophils) increase in number and become more efficient, while the number of T-cells changes and phagocytic activity is reduced around the fetus and placenta. These are most probably mechanisms to ensure that the mother's immune system does not act to reject the foreign tissue of the fetus, and there are various theories as to why this does not happen. The placenta is seen as a barrier. However, fetal cells do enter the maternal circulation and are not recognised by the mother's immune system as invaders. Clearly, therefore, there is a selective immunosuppressive response.[1] Generally the increase in the number of B-cells and the decrease in the number of T-cells leaves the pregnant woman susceptible to viral infections, but capable of continuing (except around the fetus) to combat bacteria effectively.

The presence of pathogenic micro-organisms in the body is called infection, but the extent to which it is manifested is controlled by the immune system. This may mean that there is only a sub-clinical response, or the individual may maintain a 'carrier' status. However, if the pathogenic micro-organisms successfully harm cells (or the immune system's response damages tissues) then disease occurs although, depending on the site, little damage will usually be caused unless it successfully spreads to other parts of the body.[1] Many micro-organisms live in the body, some potentially pathogenic types existing without causing any damage (these are described as commensal), and others actually being beneficial (described as symbiotic).

As the immune system has evolved to deal with infection, the elements that cause infection have also developed many characteristics in an attempt to try and escape detection by the immune system. Some micro-organisms live within cells (e.g. HIV lives in the immune system's cells, and the malaria parasite lives in red blood cells and liver cells) and thus hide from the immune system. Some invading micro-organisms can change the proteins on their surface to make it difficult for the immune system to recognise them.[2]

The body is protected by both an innate (natural) immune system and an adaptive (acquired) immune system, which are interconnected and will function as soon as there is a need for them, as well as over a more prolonged period.

Innate system

The innate system (also termed natural, non-inducible or constitutive) is non-specific, but includes the components listed in Box 2.1.

Box 2.1   Components of the innate system

- Barriers
- Phagocytes
- Natural killer cells
- Complement system

Barriers

Skin

The most basic defence is unbroken skin, which provides both a physical and a chemical barrier. The skin, which is continuous with the mucosa (which lines the external openings of the body and has its own specific defences) is the largest organ of the body and can weigh up to 5 kg in an adult. Skin is physically tough and resists injury. Together with additional structures such as hair, which can cushion vulnerable areas (e.g. the head), it provides a mechanical barrier. Secretions such as sweat and sebum contain substances (e.g. lactic acid and free fatty acids) which inhibit microbial growth. Lactic acid in particular, by creating an environment with a low pH, inhibits many pathogenic micro-organisms. The skin also has normal bacterial flora growing on it, which can successfully compete for space and nutrients with pathogenic bacteria and fungi.

The skin consists of several layers.

- The *epidermis* is avascular and is composed of squamous epithelial cells or keratinocytes. It is divided into sub-layers.
- The *basement membrane* (or dermo-epidermal junction) is the area that separates the epidermis from the dermis.
- The *dermis* is the thickest skin layer. It contains fibroblasts that synthesise collagen (which provides strength) and elastin (which provides the ability to stretch and recoil).
- The *hypodermis* is the subcutaneous layer below the dermis.

The skin is constantly experiencing a changing environment (hot, cold, wet, dry), and can be exposed to assaults of varying severity. Many complex processes maintain the skin's integrity.

It is worth noting that midwives breach this basic defence routinely (e.g. when taking blood), and often may not consider the possible consequences. Serious infection following such simple procedures is rare (although not unknown), but even small wounds may be colonised by invading bacteria,

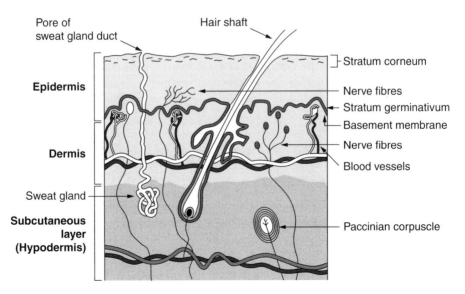

Figure 2.1 The different layers of the skin.

resulting in an immune system response. This may successfully ensure that there is no systemic infection, but will use up maternal resources which, following childbirth or in early pregnancy (when nutrition may be limited by nausea and vomiting), may not be at their optimum. Therefore basic asepsis, even when performing common routine procedures, should always be maintained.

Mucous membrane

The mucous membrane is a chemical barrier that continually produces and secretes *mucus* – a sticky, tenacious substance which can prevent bacteria from adhering to epithelial cells. Some mucous membranes (e.g. in the nose) contain *ciliated cells* that can act like a brush to move bacteria and particles that are trapped in the mucus, and thus expel it. Mucous membrane also contains IgA antibodies which can adhere to micro-organisms and prevent them from gaining access to cells, thereby stopping replication.

Other body fluids

Other body fluids, such as tears, sweat, intestinal secretions, urine and vaginal secretions, contain enzymes or antibacterial peptides, or else create a low pH that slows down or prevents bacterial invasion. Lysozyme is a specific enzyme that can attack and break down bacterial cell walls, leading to the destruction of bacteria. It is found in breast milk as well as in other body fluids. Body reflexes such as sneezing, coughing or 'watering' eyes can then rid the body of bacteria.

However, despite all of the complex external barrier systems that are present, pathogens can and do overcome these obstacles, although they do not necessarily cause disease.

Phagocytes, natural killer cells and the complement system

The next line of defence consists of phagocytic cells (also known as granu-locytes), neutrophils, eosinophils and basophils (also known as leucocytes or white blood cells), natural killer cells and the complement system of proteins. It must be noted that all of these elements overlap in terms of functions not only with each other, but also with other systems, and indeed in some cases with the acquired immune system.

Box 2.2   Normal white blood cell counts ($\times 10^9$/litre) in non-pregnant adults[3]

Neutrophils	2.0–7.0
Eosinophils	0.02–0.5
Basophils	0.02–0.1
Lymphocytes	1.0–3.0
Monocytes	0.2–1.0

Phagocytes

Phagocytosis is the process of ingesting and destroying micro-organisms. Many cells are capable of phagocytosis, but the main ones are the mononuclear phagocytes, in particular macrophages (see below) and the polymorphonuclear neutrophil leucocytes (PMN). *Neutrophils* are the most plentiful circulating phagocytes, and although they only live for a short time, they are very efficient at killing bacteria and fungi. They circulate in the blood and respond to local invasion by micro-organisms by moving into the infected tissues and destroying foreign organisms. After it has engulfed a micro-organism (intracellular killing) the neutrophil usually dies, and these dead cells are the major component of pus. Neutrophils have a vital role in wound healing (*see* Chapter 3), and are the first type of cell to appear at an inflammatory site.

Eosinophils (or oesinophils) are related to neutrophils and are specialised for killing parasites that are too large to be phagocytosed by other cells (extracellular killing).[2] They also have a role in combating antigen–antibody complexes and in influencing allergic reactions.[4]

Basophils are also related to neutrophils but are not capable of phagocytosis. They produce histamine, which is involved in the inflammatory response. They help to increase the permeability of the vascular system during inflammation, as well as causing vasodilation, and thus they are an important component of wound healing (*see* Chapter 3). Basophils are capable of a hypersensitivity response and can cause symptoms of allergy. They are similar to mast cells.

Mast cells are related to neutrophils but are more specialised. They can increase vascular permeability and present antigens to the lymphocytes. Mast cells are found beneath the mucosal surface of the body and in connective tissue. They secrete many cytokines which regulate the immune response, and they are also responsible for most of the interactions between the innate and adaptive systems.[5] Mast cells orchestrate the defence against parasites and recruit eosinophils and basophils.

Dendritic cells share many of the characteristics of mast cells, but their main role is to identify the foreign pathogen for the lymphocytes. When immature, dendritic cells can enter infected tissue, taking up pathogens and concentrating them on their surface membrane. They then migrate via the lymphatic system to lymph nodes, where the resident lymphocytes can deal with the pathogens. When mature, dendritic cells can activate antigen-specific naïve T-cells. Dendritic cells also secrete many cytokines.[5]

Box 2.3   Cytokines

Cytokines (previously known as lymphokines) are glycoproteins released by various cells of the immune system (e.g. natural killer cells, lymphocytes, etc.) which stimulate activity. These include interferons (which restrict the spread of intravascular viruses), interleukins (which influence the differentiation of immune system cells) and chemokines (which are responsible for cell movement).

Cytokines are protein molecules (more than 100 different ones have been identified) produced by cells. They have many and varied functions, but are largely communication molecules.[5] If a substance affects the immunological activity of a cell it is called a cytokine.

Cytokines released by tissue phagocytic cells induce fever.[1] Pyrexia is part of the body's defence system, as by increasing the body temperature some pathogens may be killed. However, too high a temperature may damage enzymes and normal cellular processes.

Natural killer cells

Although natural killer (NK) cells are lymphocytes (which are part of the acquired immune system), they have no antigen-specific receptors and are usually considered to be part of the innate system. NK cells are large granular lymphocytes which develop in the bone marrow and circulate in the blood and lymph.

When a vulnerable cell recognises a virus, it can produce *interferons* which inhibit pathogen replication and activate NK cells. Interferons are one of the antimicrobial agents that exhibit a non-specific response to infection, and they supplement the NK cytotoxicity.[6] The interferon can bind to specific receptors on uninfected cells and protect them from the virus, thereby limiting the spread of the virus. Interferon may also inhibit the division of viruses inside cells.[2]

NK cells can also be activated by macrophage-derived cytokines. The NK cells target and destroy some virus-infected cells as well as the cells of some types of tumours. In pregnancy, NK activity is restricted around the uterus and therefore pregnant women's response to pathogens such as *Listeria* or *Toxoplasma* may be compromised.[7]

Complement system

The complement system is a complex system consisting of more than 20 proteins that react together. It is activated by pathogens or IgM and IgG antibodies, and it initiates the inflammatory response, increases the permeability of tissues to blood plasma proteins and facilitates phagocytosis, helping to restrict the spread of infecting micro-organisms.

Monocyte–macrophage system (formerly called reticulo-endothelial system)

Mononuclear phagocytes occur both in blood (where they are called monocytes) and in tissues (where they are called macrophages). This system includes the tissues where macrophages are most common, such as the liver, spleen, kidney, lungs and lymph nodes, all of which have large numbers of macrophages and therefore provide filtration of blood and lymph.[2] However, macrophages can also be found in all other body tissues.

Macrophages engulf bacteria and then digest them by the process of phagocytosis. They also produce toxic substances that help to kill the engulfed micro-organisms, and these substances can also destroy some other parasites by extracellular killing (cytotoxicity). The interaction between the pathogen and tissue macrophage, leading to the release of cytokines, also induces inflammation, which brings neutrophils and plasma proteins to the site.[1]

> Macrophages and mast cells represent the front line of defence and initiate inflammation.

Adaptive system

The adaptive system (which may also be described as acquired or inducible) is the second immune response and is specific against a particular organism.

After the initial exposure, the immune system usually reacts more quickly to subsequent exposures, and this response time is usually shortened by repeated infection.

An example of a situation in which this heightened response is undesirable is rhesus isoimmunisation, where in the first pregnancy of a rhesus-negative mother carrying a rhesus-positive fetus, the mother's immune system will react slowly to the rhesus-positive fetal cells in her system. However, in future pregnancies, since her immune system is already sensitised, it will react more quickly and her antibodies can cross the placenta to attack rhesus-positive fetal cells. The degree of severity can range from treatable jaundice in the neonate to the death of the fetus. Fortunately, anti-D immunoglobulin, which is now widely available, can prevent antibody production.

Box 2.4   Antigens

Antigens are foreign micro-organisms and are either proteins or sugars. An antigen can be defined as a substance that induces an immunological response in an immunocompetent individual, so it might be the whole pathogenic cell, a substance secreted by that cell or a substance produced by non-pathogenic cells (e.g. plant pollen).

The main difference between innate and adaptive immunity is that adaptive immunity is specific to an individual antigen, and after making a specific response this can lead to an altered state of immunity or memory. Therefore each person's adaptive immune system will be unique to them, depending on their past exposures.

Lymphoid system

The lymphoid system consists of primary sites where lymphocytes are produced (the bone marrow, thymus and fetal liver), and secondary sites to which the lymphocytes travel. These sites include the spleen, lymph nodes and other lymphoid tissue throughout the body (e.g. tonsils, appendix), which the lymphocytes reach via the lymphatic vessels.

Lymphocytes are cells that recognise antigens.

Lymphocytes can work in different ways. They can:

- directly destroy antigens
- secrete proteins called antibodies
- secrete substances that influence other cells (some of which regulate the actions of the lymphocytes that reacted to the original antigen).

There are two types of lymphocytes.

- **B-cells** originate and mature in the bone marrow. When activated these differentiate into plasma cells which produce antibodies (humoral immunity) or memory cells.
- **T-cells** also originate in the bone marrow, and travel to the thymus to complete their maturation process (cell-mediated immunity). They include cytotoxic or suppressor (CD8) T-cells, which regulate the destruction of cells infected with viruses, and 'helper' (CD4) T-cells, which differentiate into cells that activate other cells such as B-cells and macrophages.

Both B- and T-cells enter the bloodstream after maturation and then travel to the peripheral lymphoid organs. There are about two billion lymphocytes in an adult, and about 50% of these are associated with mucosal tissues, protecting against micro-organisms that attempt to enter the body.

Lymphocytes circulate throughout the body, between the bloodstream and secondary sites, until they encounter an antigen and become activated. Lymph nodes and other lymphoid tissue can collect antigens from the sites of infection, making them available to the lymphocytes, which have recognition systems for detecting pathogens.

Lymphocytes sense the presence of antigens by means of lymphocyte antigen receptors (immunoglobulin on B-cells and T-cell receptors on T-cells). Receptors produced by each lymphocyte have unique antigen specificity. Because the adult body contains about two billion lymphocytes, it can respond to a great variety of antigens.

B-cells

When B-cells encounter an antigen they proliferate and differentiate into memory cells or differentiated plasma cells.[8] One activated B-cell can produce about 40–100 memory cells. These memory cells can be activated by another antigen exposure and usually react faster in subsequent exposures. Activation of B-cells and differentiation into antibody-secreting plasma cells is triggered by the antigen and usually requires helper T-cells.[1]

Newly produced B-cells which become plasma cells can produce large amounts of antigen-specific antibodies for many days until they die, and these plasma cells can be produced for as long as they are needed.

B-cells also present the antigen to the T-helper cells that produce cytokines, which stimulate B-cells to continue to differentiate and produce more antibodies.

B-cells have cell-surface immunoglobulin (also called surface or membrane antibody) molecules as receptors for the antigen, and after activation they secrete the immunoglobulin (a soluble antibody that provides defence against the pathogens in extracellular spaces).

Thus antibodies are found in plasma and extracellular fluids and can act to destroy pathogens in various ways. By binding to the pathogen the antibody can neutralise it, blocking its access to cells. An antibody can also coat a pathogen so that a phagocyte can recognise it, and can sometimes enhance phagocytic action. When an antibody is bound to the antigen it is called an *immune complex.* This immune complex can also active the complement system.

Immunoglobulins are specialised glycoproteins and are divided into various classes and subclasses, depending on their structure. Immunoglobulins exist in both membrane-bound form (B-cell receptors) and secreted form (antibodies). The five main classes are as follows.

1. **IgG** circulates in tissue fluids and blood, and may block virus entry into cells and destroy viruses and bacteria. It is the most abundant immunoglobulin in body fluids, particularly extravascularly, where it combats micro-organisms and their toxins.[6] It can bind to a pathogen and promote ingestion (antibody-mediated phagocytosis). IgG memory cells are present in the body for a long time, and may therefore indicate acute infection, previous exposure or vaccination. IgG also crosses the placenta during late pregnancy and is found in the intestine of the neonate. In addition it is present in colostrum and breast milk.
2. **IgM** circulates in tissue fluids and blood. It is produced at an early stage and is an effective first-level defence against bacteria, being an efficient agglutinator. It may block virus entry into cells and can destroy viruses.[2] As it is an early response and will disappear after recovery, serum IgM is a marker of acute infection. It is the only antibody that is made by the fetus.
3. **IgA** is found primarily in sero-mucous secretions, protecting external body surfaces. Although it does not cross the placenta, it is a major immunoglobulin in breast milk, and it remains in the neonatal intestines to protect mucosal surfaces.[6]
4. **IgE** is concerned with the protection of the external body surface. Its levels are increased in parasitic infection, and it is responsible for the

symptoms of atopic allergy. Responses involve mast cell degranulation, but the symptoms differ depending on whether the allergen is ingested, inhaled or eaten, and on what dose is involved.[1]

5. **IgD** is found mainly in the blood on lymphocyte surfaces, and is probably concerned with the differentiation of lymphocytes. Its function is not known for certain, but is related to tolerance.

Antibodies cannot reach micro-organisms inside host cells. Therefore the acquired immune system evolved a further response, involving T-cells, which are specialised to work against cells containing intracellular organisms.

T-cells

A T-cell is a lymphocyte that is concerned with the control of intracellular infection – each T-cell has its own individual antigen receptor. Until the circulating T-cell encounters an antigen it is called a naive T-cell. A T-cell needs to have an antigen 'presented' to it, and three cells which can serve as antigen-presenting cells are dendritic cells, macrophages and B-cells.

Measurement of specific T-cells can give an indication of the health of the immune system. For example, a rise in CD8 levels can indicate immune system compromise. T-cell deficiencies that are acquired (e.g. AIDS) render an individual susceptible to infection caused by micro-organisms such as that responsible for tuberculosis, and by fungi, which can grow intracellularly.

> *Major histocompatibility complex* (MHC) molecules are antigen receptors. Their function is to present the pathogen to the circulating T-cells, and the T-cells can only recognise an antigen if it is presented with the MHC molecule.

Infectious agents

The four classes of infectious agents are bacteria, viruses, parasites and fungi.

Bacteria

Bacteria are single-celled organisms with the potential to cause infection. They are usually capable of independent existence, although some are parasitic.

Symbiotic bacteria often live in the urinogenitary or gastrointestinal tracts. Although they can have a protective effect, preventing pathogenic organisms from obtaining sufficient nutrients to be able to multiply, infection can occur if the balance of bacteria is disturbed (e.g. as a result of taking antibiotics).

Immunity to bacteria varies according to whether the organisms live inside or outside the cell. Although many bacteria can be repelled or even destroyed by the body's basic defences, some bacteria have developed the ability to circumvent these. For example, some bacteria (e.g. *Mycobacterium tuberculosis*) can survive and divide inside macrophages after being phagocytosed, and need T-cell activation to contain the bacterial infection. Some bacteria have a capsule which enables them to resist destruction, while others produce endotoxins which can damage neutrophils.

Pregnancy can influence the way in which the immune system deals with bacteria. There is an increase in B-cell activity, which generally makes the body very efficient in dealing with bacteria. However, there are exceptions, such as the area around the fetus and placenta, which shows reduced phagocytic activity during pregnancy. There also seems to be increased susceptibility to *Helicobacter pylori* infection in pregnancy. This bacterium can cause various abdominal symptoms as well as gastroduodenal pathology.[9]

Viruses

Viruses consist of a core of nucleic acids surrounded by a protein coat, and are the most widespread of all pathogens.

Since most viruses can only replicate intracellularly, virus destruction also causes cell destruction. If a virus can survive in a cell without destroying it, a 'carrier' state may exist, whereby an asymptomatic person can be infectious (e.g. hepatitis B). A virus can also become dormant or latent (e.g. herpes) and then become reactivated in the future, causing another acute infection, often when the immune system is stressed. Therefore pregnancy and the puerperium are vulnerable times. During pregnancy the reduction in the number of helper T-cells leaves the woman susceptible to viral infection.

Virus-infected cells may be destroyed by cytotoxic T-cells, NK cells and interferons. Two immune responses to a virus are necessary – one occurring outside the cell in the circulation during the virus's spread from cell to cell, and the other to reach intracellular viruses. Many viruses can change their surface coats and consequently specific protective immunity (or vaccine production) is not possible. For example, the influenza virus changes often, and therefore vaccine is of only limited use, whereas the smallpox virus changes little and vaccine is therefore very effective.

Parasites

There are many definitions of a parasite, but basically it can be described as any organism that lives in or on the body of others, or which obtains sustenance from them.

Parasites include protozoa (of which *Plasmodium*, responsible for malaria, is the most common), helminths (e.g. flukes) and nematodes (e.g. roundworms). Many parasites have developed mechanisms for avoiding the immune system. For example, some have the ability to hide inside cells or capsules, while others may mimic host characteristics. Parasites can produce an antibody response if they are in the bloodstream, but if they are contained within cells a T-cell response is necessary. However, long-term immunity does not always occur.

Parasitic invasion can be extremely significant in pregnant women in parts of the world where parasites are common, as the compromised immune system and/or resulting anaemia can be particularly hazardous at the time of delivery.[10]

Fungi

Fungi occur in two forms, namely single-celled yeasts and multicellular moulds.

Most fungi are harmless, and those that can affect humans are usually opportunistic – that is, they will only become a problem in individuals whose immune system is compromised or deficient. An example is candida (thrush), which often becomes apparent when antibiotics upset the balance of the normal vaginal flora.

Potential complications of the immune system

Autoimmune reaction

Some lymphocytes have the potential to react to self-antigens, but usually remain under some form of control. This is useful for wound healing, but can also lead to autoimmune disease in some individuals.[2] Despite much research, the actual cause of autoimmune disease is unknown.[5] However, it is known that women suffer more than men, and there is evidence of a genetic predisposition.[6] It is thought that autoimmunity may be triggered by an infection in genetically susceptible individuals (e.g. in cases of diabetes mellitus).

Autoimmune disease can be systemic (e.g. anti-DNA antibodies in systemic lupus erythematosus, SLE) or organ-specific (e.g. antibodies to pancreatic β-cells in insulin-dependent diabetes mellitus). In the case of SLE it is unknown why large amounts of anti-DNA antibodies are made, but they bind to DNA to form immune complexes which then lodge at various sites, such as the kidney, skin or blood–brain barrier, and lead to inflammation. Pregnancy may cause exacerbation of autoimmune diseases such as SLE, probably due to the increased activity of B-cells in pregnancy.[11] Indeed these diseases may become clinically obvious for the first time, and diagnosed, during pregnancy or in the puerperium. Some autoimmune diseases (e.g. rheumatoid arthritis) may actually improve during pregnancy.

Some autoimmune diseases may affect the newborn. In some cases the neonate will clear the maternal antibody with no ill effects. However, sometimes the neonate will need plasmapheresis to remove maternal antibodies before they can cause damage, although occasionally permanent injury may have occurred *in utero*.[1] Autoantibodies may also be present in breast milk.

Hypersensitivity

Normally when the initial immune system response to the antigen has been mounted, the system is ready to deal with the next exposure more efficiently. However, occasionally the reaction may be excessive, and this is described as hypersensitivity.[6] This may occur either because the body was exposed to excessive antigens, or because too many antibodies were produced.[2]

Hypersensitivity can be divided into five types, depending on the immunological mechanism involved.

- **Type I** (e.g. hayfever, asthma or anaphylactic hypersensitivity) is the formation of excessive IgE antibody specific for the antigen, and this can cause tissue damage.[8] Most allergies involve the production of IgE antibody to common environmental allergens,[1] and about 10% of the population suffers from allergies such as hayfever, asthma, or drug or food allergies involving localised IgE-mediated anaphylactic reactions.[6]

Anaphylaxis is the involuntary contraction of smooth muscle and dilation of capillaries, and in its extreme form can be fatal.

- **Type II** is antibody-dependent cytotoxic hypersensitivity, which involves the death of the cell bearing the antibody attached to a surface antigen – for example, transfusion reactions or haemolytic disease of the newborn (HDN) due to rhesus incompatibility.
- **Type III** is immune complex hypersensitivity, in which increased levels of antigen lead to overload and deposition in the tissues. This may eventually progress to tissue damage. Examples include farmer's lung and the various organ- and/or tissue-damaged sites in SLE.[6]
- **Type IV** is cell-mediated hypersensitivity in which T-cell or macrophagic activation persists in response to skin-sensitising or ongoing infection (e.g. contact dermatitis or leprosy).
- **Type V** is stimulatory hypersensitivity in which the antibody reacts with, for example, a hormone receptor and 'switches on' the cell (e.g. thyroid hypersensitivity in Graves' disease due to thyroid-stimulating autoantibody).[6]

Immunosuppression

The immune system can become less effective or suppressed for many reasons, including disease or treatments, the presence of a gene defect causing an inherited failure of defence, environmental factors and possibly psycho-social issues.

Immunosuppressive drugs

Following organ transplant, immunosuppressive drugs are necessary to prevent rejection of the foreign tissue, and a certain level of immunodeficiency is inevitable. Nevertheless, there is growing evidence of the possibility of a successful pregnancy following a kidney transplant[12] or liver transplant.[13] There is also increasing evidence that it may be possible to treat some pregnant women who have cancer using chemotherapy without damaging the fetus, although again some maternal immunosuppression may be present.[14]

Pathogens

Many pathogens can suppress the immune response. For example, staphylococci can lead to generalised immunosuppression. Some pathogens, such as the measles virus, may cause mild or transient immunosuppression, but can often be fatal in malnourished children if bacterial infection follows.[1]

HIV

HIV is an enveloped retrovirus that replicates in cells of the immune system, and infection with HIV causes the loss of CD4 T-cells. After the initial infection and the appearance of antibodies, the infected individual usually experiences a long asymptomatic period. However, although the person is externally apparently healthy, there are changes in the distribution of cells in the lymphoid tissue, and T-cell numbers begin to fall. As the number of CD4 T-cells fall, opportunistic infection occurs. Potential immune suppression due to HIV is of concern to midwives because of the growing number of HIV-positive women they now see. The latest evidence shows that pregnancy does not hasten the progress of HIV.[15] However, there are some adverse pregnancy outcomes that may be more common in women with HIV, such as a suggested increased risk of miscarriage, chorioamnionitis or intrauterine growth-restricted babies.[16] There does not appear to be a direct link between pregnancy complications and the drug treatment for HIV.[15]

Corticosteroids

Corticosteroids are produced by the cortex of the adrenal glands, and are natural regulators of immune cell function, altering the way in which cells travel around the body and slowing down cell division. When given as a drug, synthetic corticosteroids can cause an anti-inflammatory response and suppress the immune system.

Traumatic injury

Traumatic injury, including surgery, can be immunosuppressive because corticosteroids are produced by increased stress, immunosuppressive prostaglandin E2 is released from damaged tissues, and bacterial endotoxins are released as a result of the disturbance of the flora in the gut and reproductive system, all of which can affect the functioning of the immune system.[6] Therefore after delivery, when a woman may have greatest need of an optimum immune response, there may be elements of immunosuppression.

Malnutrition (see Chaper 4)

The immune system requires good nutrition if it is to be at its most effective, and a poor immune response occurs in cases of protein/energy malnutrition. There is also good evidence of an impaired immune response in individuals with a deficiency of pyridoxine, folic acid and vitamins A, C and E. Poor digestion and/or absorption of nutrients can also impair the working of the immune system of individuals with parasites or malabsorption disease.

In addition, there is some evidence that pollution in the food chain may influence immunity.[6]

Exercise

Extreme exercise can lead to reduced IgA levels, immunodeficiency and increased susceptibility to infection.[6] However, exercise is much more likely to form part of a healthy lifestyle and a strong immune system – this is just a reminder that extremes in most things can lead to undesirable outcomes.

Sex hormones

Oestrogen is the main factor influencing the more active immune response in women compared with that in men. Women have increased serum IgG and secreted IgA levels, an increased antibody response to T-cell-independent antigens and greater resistance to infection. However, they also exhibit increased susceptibility to autoimmune disease (see above).

Environmental/social factors

Environmental effects such as pollution can play a part in suppressing the immune system. A study that was conducted in the Czech Republic compared two groups of women and found that mothers from a district known to be highly polluted had a lower percentage of total T-cells and in particular CD4 cells, and there was also a lower percentage of T-cells and an increased percentage of NK cells in cord blood taken from the newborns at birth.[17]

Alcohol consumption and smoking are associated with changes in a number of immune parameters, and these variations can be measured in breast milk.[18] Smoking is known to depress the immune system. It also specifically interferes with wound healing (see Chapters 3 and 4). Smoking during pregnancy is known to be related to poor outcomes both for the pregnancy and for the neonate.[19] However, midwives need to work closely with smoking cessation professionals and others to give these women optimum support. Often smoking is only one aspect of the woman's problems,[20] and may indeed be the only way she has of coping with stress.

Stress

An increase in glucocorticoid levels is a major response to stresses induced by a wide range of stimuli (e.g. fear, physical injury, etc.).[4] If cortisol levels remain elevated (e.g. in response to chronic stress), the number of white blood cells falls, the number of lymphocytes decreases and there is a less efficient immune system response. The production of cytokines may also be inhibited.[21]

Stress has been commonly associated with preterm birth, and it has been suggested that one possible explanation for this may be that the maternal immune system becomes suppressed, thereby increasing susceptibility to intrauterine and fetal infections and the inflammatory processes.[22] Therefore it has been suggested that reducing stressors which lead to physiological changes can decrease the incidence of preterm labour.[23]

It has also been suggested that psychosocial stress during pregnancy can cause maternal immunosuppression, which may lead to other pregnancy complications and influence fetal development.[24]

With its vital range of influence over the well-being of a pregnant woman or new mother, the importance of a healthy immune system cannot be over-emphasised. The challenge for midwives will be to find interventions that can support or improve the immune system in a way that is tailored to each individual woman's need.

References

1 Janeway C, Travers P, Walport M *et al.* (2001) *Immunobiology: the immune system in health and disease* (5e). Garland Publishing, New York.

2 Staines N, Brostoff J and James K (1993) *Introducing Immunology* (2e). Mosby, London.

3 Dacie J and Lewis S (1995) *Practical Haematology* (8e). Churchill Livingstone, London.

4 Bray J, Cragg P, MacKnight A *et al.* (1999) *Lecture Notes on Human Physiology* (4e). Blackwell Publishing, Oxford.

5 Playfair J and Bancroft G (2004) *Infection and Immunity* (2e). Oxford University Press, Oxford.

6 Roitt I (1997) *Roitt's Essential Immunology* (9e). Blackwell Science, Oxford.

7 Wegman T, Lin H, Guilbert L *et al.* (1993) Bi-directional cytokine interactions in the maternal–fetal relationship: is successful pregnancy a TH2 phenomenon? *Immunol Today.* **15:** 15–18.

8 Kreir J and Mortensen R (1990) *Infection, Resistance and Immunity.* Harper & Row Publishers, New York.

9 Lanciers S, Despinasse B, Mehta D *et al.* (1999) Increased susceptibility to *Helicobacter pylori* infection in pregnancy. *Infect Dis Obstet Gynecol.* **7:** 195–8.

10 Harrison K (2001) Anaemia in pregnancy. In: J Lawson, K Harrison and S Bergstrom (eds) *Maternal Care in Developing Countries.* RCOG Press, London.

11 Coad J (2001) *Anatomy and Physiology for Midwives.* Mosby, Edinburgh.

12 Marsh J, Maclean D and Pattison J (2001) Renal disease: best practice and research. *Clin Obstet Gynaecol.* **15:** 891–901.

13 Gandhi H and Davies N (2004) Liver transplants and obstetrics. *J Obstet Gynaecol.* **24:** 771–3.

14 Cardonick E and Iacobucci A (2004) Use of chemotherapy during human pregnancy. *Lancet.* **5:** 283–91.

15 Pratt R (2003) *HIV and AIDS: a foundation for nursing and healthcare practices* (5e). Arnold, London.

16 French R and Brocklehurst P (1998) The effects of pregnancy on survival in women infected with HIV: a systematic review of the literature and meta-analysis. *Br J Obstet Gynaecol.* **105:** 827–35.

17 Hertz-Picciotto I, Dostal M, Dejmek J *et al.* (2002) Air pollution and distribution of lymphocyte immunophenotypes in cord and maternal blood at delivery. *Epidemiology.* **13:** 172–83.

18 Na H, Daniels L and Seelig L (1997) Preliminary study of how alcohol consumption during pregnancy affects immune components in breast milk and blood of postpartum women. *Alcohol Alcoholism.* **32:** 581–9.

19 Tobacco Information Campaign (2002) Helping pregnant women to stop smoking. *Br J Midwifery.* **10:** 663–6.

20 Allen H (2000) Helping pregnant smokers quit – a review for health professionals. *Prof Care Mother Child.* **10:** 709–22.

21 Thomas P (2002) Stress: poison by slow motion. *What Doctors Don't Tell You.* **13:** 1–4.

22 Wadhwa R, Cukhane J, Rauh V *et al.* (2001) Stress and preterm birth: neuroendocrine, immune/inflammatory and vascular mechanisms. *Matern Child Health J.* **5:** 119–25.

23 Ruiz R and Pearson A (1999) Psychoneuroimmunology and preterm birth: a holistic model for obstetrical nursing practice and research. *MCN Am J Matern Child Nurs.* **24:** 230–5.

24 Coussons-Read M, Okun M and Simms S (2003) The psychoneuroimmunology of pregnancy. *J Reprod Infant Psychol.* **21:** 103–12.

3

Wound healing

Wound healing is the process of replacement and restoration of function of damaged tissues.[1]

For the new mother, many of the normal physical components of the postnatal period involve healing to some degree. The puerperium is generally considered to include the return of the woman's body to its non-pregnant state, and much of the process is concerned with involution of the uterus, together with healing of the placental site (itself a large 'wound') involving ischaemia and autolysis. The successful resolution of this is vital for the woman's health, but apart from nutritional guidance (which should ideally have been given during the antenatal period) and basic advice about hygiene and lifestyle, there is little that the midwife can do to influence this process.

However, other wounds are also very common following childbirth, and the midwife has a key role in giving advice and care with regard to them. Perineal wounds affect about 75% of women following a vaginal birth, and of course are more likely after an instrumental delivery. Caesarean section wounds are also becoming an increasingly common part of a midwife's responsibility,[2] and despite much effort it seems unlikely these numbers will decline significantly. Both of these types of traumatic wound fall clearly within the midwife's remit, with her accountability for the care of women during the postnatal period.[3]

Resources for midwives in relation to detailed wound care are not immediately obvious. The traditional midwifery texts include little on the theory of wound healing and care. With an increasing number of 'direct-entry' midwives who have not had previous experience of nursing wounds, it is clear that in order to undertake effective care, midwives will need to access specialist material in order to keep up to date.

Assessment and care of perineal and Caesarean section wounds are such an important part of the midwife's role that care issues with regard to these wounds warrant specific analysis. This can be found in Chapter 5 (on perineal wounds) and Chapter 6 (on Caesarean section wounds). However, under-pinning all good wound care is the theory of wound healing, and it may be seen as important for a midwife to have an understanding of this process on which to base her care. This chapter can of course only give an overview, but the reference list at the end may provide a starting point for those who wish to delve into this fascinating area in more detail.

Stages of wound healing

The biology of wound healing is less than 100 years old and this new science is continually developing.[4] All actions in wound healing are regulated by a complex series of chemical reactions which initiate, control or inhibit various factors, and all of these actions are interrelated. However, although many actions overlap, for the purposes of explanation the stages can be divided as follows.

Immediate reactions: vasoconstriction/ activation of clotting, platelets and endothelial cells/haemostasis/ clot formation

Immediately after an injury the blood vessels constrict around the site, and this vasoconstriction leads to a rapid reduction in bleeding. The cellular disruption exposes blood to air, and this helps to activate the coagulation process.[5] Platelets attach themselves to the exposed sub-endothelium of the injury and clump together (a process termed aggregation), and together with fibrin (a blood protein) form a clot, filling the space of the injury and bringing the sides together. The fibrin clot consists mainly of red blood cells, but can also incorporate dead tissue or even foreign matter.

Inflammation

An acute inflammatory response occurs within hours of the injury, and its effect can last for 5 to 7 days. Tissue damage and the resulting activation of clotting factors cause the release of various vasoactive substances, such as prosta-glandins and histamine, which lead to increased vasodilation and increased permeability of the blood vessels as well as stimulation of pain fibres.[6]

First-line defence: leucocytes.
Second-line defence: monocytes.

The fibrin clot attracts leucocytes,[7] and within the first 24 hours specifically neutrophils (which attack and remove bacteria and damaged cells) and monocytes (scavenger cells – once in the tissue these are called macrophages) appear. Neutrophils ingest and kill foreign material and in the process of doing so many of these cells die. In infection, these dead cells and other waste matter are the constituents of pus.[8]

Macrophages play an important part in most phases of wound healing, not only in clearing the wound site but also in producing growth factors and other substances that control the processes. New capillaries begin to grow into the wound (angiogenesis), resulting (most importantly) in the formation of a new connective tissue matrix.[9]

Vasodilation not only enables neutrophils and monocytes to be easily delivered to the site, but also results in the production of exudate which may lead to oedema. There is leakage of serous fluid into the wound bed, and normal wound healing requires the growth factors, nutrients and bacterial activity factors that are present in this inflammatory exudate.[10] However, depending on the location of the wound, the pressure of even a slight amount of excess fluid/oedema may cause some pain, as in the case of perineal wounds.

Depending on the wound's position, the increase in blood flow may cause the area to appear red in colour. The vasodilation and additional metabolic activity can also produce heat, so that the area feels warm to the touch.

Normal inflammation is therefore characterised by the following:

- redness (erythema)
- possibly some swelling
- a slight local increase in temperature (or in the case of a large wound, systemic pyrexia)
- possibly some pain.

However, any exaggeration of these signs may indicate infection (see later in this chapter).

During the transition from the inflammatory phase to the proliferative phase, the number of inflammatory cells declines and the number of fibroblasts increases.

Proliferation: reconstruction/granulation (angiogenesis/collagen production/ epithelialisation/contraction)

During the proliferation phase, new blood vessels continue to form throughout the wound (angiogenesis or neovascularisation). This process is vital, as no new tissue can be built without new blood vessels supplying oxygen and nutrients. Angiogenic growth factors secreted by macrophages (probably in response to the tissue hypoxia) stimulate the endothelium to divide and organise the growth of the new blood vessels. Intact vessels around the wound 'bud' new vessels which spread throughout the wound and multiply.

Macrophages appear to need less oxygen than other cells, and can therefore move further into the wound.[8] As they divide within the wound site to kill microbes and clear dead tissue, the increase in the number of macrophages also attracts fibroblasts (cells that produce collagen – a primary protein of connective tissue that provides the latter with strength).

Fibroblasts proliferate from about 2 to 4 days after injury, and produce a matrix (a scaffold-like structure) of collagen around the new vessels. They are stimulated to produce collagen by lactate and ascorbate (a form of ascorbic acid), which are present in the hypoxic wound bed.[11] The fibroblasts move over the matrix, granulation tissue (including fibroblasts, collagen, new blood vessels and macrophages) proliferates and epithelialisation (the migration of epidermal cells over the surface) occurs, commencing restoration of the epithelial barrier functions of the skin.[9]

The epidermis is a multi-layer epithelium consisting of epidermal cells (*see* Chapter 2 for a more detailed description of the skin). Epithelial cells migrate either as a complete moving sheet or by 'leap-frogging' over viable tissue. Epithelial cells cannot move across a dry surface or necrotic tissue, so an open wound needs to be full of granulation tissue before epithelialisation can take place. The presence of 'crusting' or scabs also forms a barrier to epithelial cells, and they are forced to burrow underneath this.[5] In ideal conditions, wound epithelialisation may occur within 48–72 hours.[12]

Also contributing to the wound closure is the contraction of the wound edges, which decreases the size of the wound by the work of the myofibroblasts.[7] Contraction does not occur in surgical wounds, which are immediately sutured, as it is unnecessary because they require minimal collagen synthesis and little epidermal cell migration to cover the deficit.

Maturation: remodelling

The initial fibrin clot is replaced by granulation tissue which, after it has expanded until it fills the defect and has become covered by a viable epidermal surface, undergoes remodelling. This usually occurs about 20 days after injury, although the timing can vary according to individual circumstances. During remodelling the density of macrophages and fibroblasts decreases, the growth of capillaries stops and blood flow and metabolic activity decrease. Also during remodelling the excess collagen is removed and the original collagen is gradually replaced with stronger and more highly organised collagen that is laid down in a more orderly fashion along the lines of mechanical stress, although it is never as well organised as the original.[11] The remodelling phase begins at different times within different areas of the wound, and this can continue for up to a year or even longer. Thus although the wound may superficially appear to be healed, the rebuilding process continues below.[9] Remodelled tissue is never as strong as the original, and at best has been reported to have about 80% of the strength of non-wounded tissue.[11]

Scars

The remodelling of granulation tissue may be the most important contributor to problems developing from scarring. During remodelling the density of the fibroblasts decreases and they mature into a scar. The epidermis of a scar is different to that of normal skin. After healing it is thick compared with that of undamaged skin, but not as thick as that of freshly closed wounds.[9] Hair follicles and sebaceous or sweat glands do not regenerate in the scar.

The dermis of a healed wound is also different, as the arrangement of the organised collagen-fibre bundles may be altered. The degree of disruption is dependent on factors such as the location of the wound, as well as inherited factors. The healed quality of the scar can vary in terms of appearance, size and whether full function is restored. A Caesarean section scar needs to be strong in order to deal with stresses such as support, weight gain and exercise, whereas a perineal scar needs to be flat and pliable in order to maximise comfort.

Some wounds may heal but do not result in an acceptable scar. *Hypertrophic scars* consist of an increase in tissue produced by enlargement of the existing cells. Although prominent, such a scar will remain within the boundaries of the original wound. These scars may resolve in time.

Keloid scars are usually red or brown in colour, prominent and possibly painful or itchy. They often occur some time after the injury, and are probably due to an increase in collagen synthesis. There may be a link with melanocyte-stimulating hormone, as keloid scars are most common in individuals with pigmented skin. Keloid scars are often larger than the wound, and if treated by excision they may return.[7] Treatment is usually by injection of steroids. Keloid scars have been observed following Caesarean section, but perineal keloid scars are extremely unusual.

Dehiscence is the opening of surgically closed wounds, and it may involve only part of the skin layer or the entire wound, including exposure of the abdominal organs.[13] It usually occurs if for some reason the wound is not strong enough to withstand the forces that are placed on it – a wound is at risk of dehiscence if there is infection or haematomas. The dehiscence of a previous uterine scar during labour is of particular concern to midwives.

Surgical wounds may open for the following reasons:

- infection
- increasing fluid levels (e.g. haematoma)
- the presence of a foreign body
- an underlying disease process.

How wounds heal

Wounds can heal by *primary intention*, which occurs when wound edges are brought together (approximated) by suturing. When a wound is sutured, there is a close approximation of the tissues and no 'dead space'. Therefore there is minimal granulation tissue necessary and contraction has a minor role. The epithelium will migrate over the suture line, and healing is primarily by connective tissue deposition.

Healing by *secondary intention* (where there is a tissue deficit) requires the formation of granulation tissue and wound contraction. This can result in increased amounts of dense, fibrous scar tissue, and such healing also takes longer.

It is clear when these points are considered that accurate assessment of perineal tears is vital when deciding whether or not to suture (*see* Chapter 5). If the perineal wound is not approximated and/or if there is a tissue deficit that will result in a 'dead space', there will be healing by secondary intent with increased granulation and the possibility of increased scar formation, as well as a longer healing time.

Wounds that have broken down often have the wound edges left open and heal 'from the bottom up' by means of granulation tissue and wound contraction (secondary intention). In midwifery care, this normally only occurs with a broken down (with or without infection) perineal wound, although recent research may not support this practice (*see* Chapter 5). Rarely, a broken down Caesarean section wound may be left to heal by secondary intention, although healing by third intention is more common.

A delayed primary repair (or healing by *third intention*) occurs when a contaminated wound is initially kept open by packing, allowing a good inflammatory response and the increased growth of new vessels at the edge of the wound. After a few days, the packing is removed and the wound is sutured.[9]

Potential barriers to successful wound healing

Box 3.1   Influences on wound healing

Tissue perfusion and oxygen
Smoking
Sleep deprivation
Stress
Medical conditions and treatments
Nutritional status
Infection
Sub-optimum care
Obesity

Although specific risks to perineal and Caesarean section wounds will be discussed in Chapters 5 and 6, there are many general factors which may compromise effective wound healing, and several of these may apply to new mothers.

Malnutrition

Malnutrition in general can lead to reduced strength of the wound, increased wound dehiscence and increased susceptibility to infection and poor-quality scarring. Specific nutrient deficiencies can have an effect on healing. For example, zinc deficiency reduces rates of epithelialisation, reduces collagen synthesis and therefore reduces wound strength. Essential unsaturated fatty acids (*see* Chapter 4) are involved in the inflammatory phase, and fat is a component of cell membranes. Vitamin A is important in cell differentiation and epithelial keratinisation, and a deficiency will lead to collagen deficiency and delayed epithelialisation. In addition, vitamin A deficiency increases susceptibility to infection. Vitamin C is also important, as collagen formed without adequate vitamin C is weaker. Several B vitamins, iron, zinc, copper and manganese all make significant contributions. Obesity, which can mask an impaired nutritional state, is known to be a risk factor for success in wound healing.[14] (*See* Chapter 4 for a full discussion of the role of nutrition in wound healing.)

Smoking

Nicotine and carbon monoxide are known to have a damaging influence on wound healing,[15] and even limited smoking can reduce the peripheral blood flow. Smoking also reduces the levels of vitamin C, which is vital for healing.

Lack of sleep

Sleep disturbances may inhibit wound healing, as sleep encourages anabolism (the synthesis of complex molecules from simple ones), and wound healing includes anabolic processes. It would be very rare to find a new mother who enjoyed her full quota of sleep every night. Therefore all midwifery clients are at risk.

Stress

It is thought that anxiety and stress can affect the immune system and thereby inhibit wound healing.[15] Childbirth is a major life stressor, and since it is unlikely that this situation will ever change, it means that ways of supporting the immune system at this time should be identified and encouraged. Additional stress can be caused by pain, fear and sometimes narcosis, and the resulting secretion of hormones (especially norepinephrine) can lead to vascular changes that result in a reduction in oxygen levels in the tissue.[16] Increased secretion of corticosteroids can inhibit the production and functioning of leucocytes.[17] However, good supportive midwifery care at this vulnerable time may go some way towards alleviating this process.

Medical conditions and therapies

Various medical conditions can influence a woman's wound-healing ability. Immunocompromise due to sepsis or malnutrition, specific diseases such as AIDS, renal or hepatic disease or drugs such as corticosteroids can lead to a compromised ability to regulate growth factors and inflammatory and proliferative cells for wound repair.

Tissue hypoxia due to peripheral vascular disease is unlikely in childbearing women, but hypovolaemia, hypothermia and vasoconstriction can all limit the oxygen supply to tissues and may occur in a woman who has had traumatic labour experiences such as a postpartum haemorrhage. Anaemia can also impair wound healing, as red blood cells are necessary to transport oxygen to the tissues.

Tissue hypoxia, whether due to long-term medical causes, an acute situation or stress, is difficult to quantify because it can occur before measurable parameters (blood pressure, pulse, temperature or urinary output) change, and when arterial oxygen levels are adequate.[16] The first indication of tissue hypoxia may be a poorly healing wound. However, a skilled midwife can anticipate the potential problem and by ensuring that the woman is well hydrated, warm, pain-free and nutritionally maintained, as well as psychologically supported, may prevent this complication.

In diabetic women, angiopathic changes (which result in impaired perfusion) may cause a delay in wound healing. Furthermore, the inflammatory response, fibroblast proliferation and collagen deposition can be impaired in the presence of high glucose levels. Since historically diabetic women have been more likely to have Caesarean sections, and may have trouble regulating their insulin regime following surgery, the importance of avoiding hyperglycaemia in order to enable effective healing must be emphasised.

Sub-optimal care

Various activities that are undertaken by carers can inhibit efficient wound healing. The swabbing or cleaning of wounds can result in organisms being redistributed around the area, cotton wool or gauze shedding fibres into granulating tissue,[18] and disruption of newly formed tissues. The presence of foreign bodies (even as small as a hair) in a wound can cause a sinus-type wound.[19]

Optimum environment for healing

> The most effective environment for successful wound healing is moist and warm.

Since the 1960s it has been accepted that the optimum environment for wound healing is moist and warm.[20,21] Exposed wounds usually form a thick crust, and crusted wounds epithelialise more slowly than covered wounds, and therefore often require more time and metabolic activity to heal.[12] This is perhaps why perineal wounds tend to heal rapidly, although they are uncovered, as the woman's anatomy ensures that the temperature remains constant and the perineal area is usually somewhat moist.

Efficient wound healing during the regenerative phase depends on a stable moist environment.[22] A moist environment also results in less infection,[23] and there is some evidence that it reduces wound pain.[24]

Warmth is the other component required for optimum healing, as it encourages the necessary leucocyte activity.[25] The ideal wound temperature is 37°C, and a lower temperature may inhibit the activity of cells involved in the healing process.[26] Although baths or showers may certainly benefit a new mother in many ways, exposure of the wound to temperature fluctuations may compromise healing.[27] Pathogens in hospital, especially in baths or bidets, may also put a woman with an exposed wound at risk of infection[28] (*see* Chapter 9 for a discussion of the midwife's role in reducing this risk).

A wound produces exudate until epithelialisation is complete. This can be seen as a yellow stain on a dressing and is a normal part of the healing process. The exudate contains many substances that enhance healing,[12] and is vital for the formation of granulation tissue and for activating growth factors. It has also been shown that the white blood cells in exudate kill bacteria and thereby reduce infection.[29]

Infection

Box 3.2   Signs and symptoms of infection

- Increasing erythema – especially spreading cellulitis
- Increasing swelling
- Change in the volume, colour or odour of exudate
- Increasing white blood cell count
- Increasing tenderness or pain
- Pyrexia and tachycardia
- Generalised malaise

Infection can delay wound healing and give rise to increased granulation and scar tissue formation.

Wound infection involves a prolonged and modified inflammatory action. With mild symptoms there can easily be confusion between the normal inflammatory response and a response to invasive organisms. It is often difficult to tell whether a wound is *contaminated* (organisms are present in exudates but not multiplying or entering tissues), *colonised* (organisms are multiplying but without systemic reaction) or *infected* (systemic symptoms as well as spreading cellulitis)[30] (*see* Chapters 5 and 6 for a further discussion of specific perineal or Caesarean section wound infection).

Wound swabs

Wound swabs need to be taken without contamination by skin flora. Swabbing a doubtful wound may also not always give a clear answer. All open wounds are contaminated, but only an excessive amount of bacteria (>100 000 gram of tissue) indicates that there is a significant likelihood of infection.[13] However, it should be noted that beta-haemolytic streptococcus can compromise healing at levels of less than 100 000 ml.[16]

It has been suggested that without evidence of systemic infection, a report showing the presence of bacteria in the wound bed should not result in antibiotic treatment.[9] Even when there is extensive contamination, it has been noted that wounds usually heal without infection in women with normal immune system function. Therefore it would seem that a midwife would be most effective in teaching and supporting a woman in maintaining a healthy immune system and wound repair response, to ensure her optimum health, so that she can avoid unnecessary antibiotic treatment (*see* Chapter 8 for a discussion of antibiotic-resistant infections).

Wound care: past, present and future

A wound should be left undisturbed unless there is necrotic tissue or excessive exudate, which can impede healing.[31] If cleaning is necessary, it should be undertaken by irrigation – using a prepacked single-use irrigation device or a 35-ml syringe and 19-gauge needle for the ideal pressure[32] – rather than being wiped with gauze or other material which, as mentioned earlier, can traumatise the healthy tissue.[27]

Specific care of perineal wounds (*see* Chapter 5) and Caesarean section wounds (*see* Chapter 6) is discussed elsewhere, but it is interesting to consider some general issues concerning wound care, from the historical to the future.

It has long been recognised that wounds should be closed, and there is evidence of thorns, metal pins and needles with various 'threads', including cotton, silk, linen and even women's hair, being used since ancient times. A great improvement in stitching was made when the 'swaged' or 'crimped' needle was invented, so that a traumatic needle 'eye' and double thread was not necessary. Furthermore, treating natural suture material (e.g. catgut) or using synthetics reduced tissue reactions.

The covering of wounds is historic, perhaps to keep out 'ill humours'.[4] There is even evidence that 'prolonged covering of open contaminated wounds and compound fractures ... can result in successful healing'.[4] We now know that the main function of dressings is to promote rapid tissue repair by providing the ideal healing environment – warm and moist – and to protect the wound from potentially harmful agents and re-injury.

In the future, adhesives or 'superglues', which have been in use for many years for skin closure, may become more widespread in maternity use. A promising trial has been undertaken of perineal skin closure, comparing histoacryl with chromic catgut, but more evidence is needed.[33]

References

1 Tortora G and Grabowski S (1996) *Principles of Anatomy and Physiology* (8e). Harper Collins College Publications, New York.

2 Boyle M (2001) Caesarean section wound management: a challenge for midwives. *Pract Midwife.* **4:** 20–2.

3 Nursing and Midwifery Council (2004) *Midwives' Rules and Standards.* Nursing and Midwifery Council, London.

4 Leaper D (1998) History of wound healing. In: D Leaper and K Harding (eds) *Wounds: biology and management.* Oxford Medical Publications, Oxford.

5 Flanagan M (2000) The physiology of wound healing. *J Wound Care.* **9:** 299–300.

6 Bray J, Cragg P, MacKnight A *et al.* (1999) *Lecture Notes on Human Physiology* (4e). Blackwell Publishing, Oxford.

7 Bale S and Jones V (1997) *Wound Care Nursing: a patient-centred approach.* Bailliere Tindall, London.

8 Bennett G and Moody M (1995) *Wound Care for Health Professionals.* Chapman & Hall, London.

9 Iocono J, Ehrlich H, Gottrup F *et al.* (1998) The biology of healing. In: D Leaper and K Harding (eds) *Wounds: biology and management.* Oxford Medical Publications, Oxford.

10 Chen W, Rogers A and Lydon M (1992) Characterization of biologic properties of wound fluid collected during early stages of wound healing. *J Invest Dermatol.* **99:** 559–64.

11 Doughty D (1992) Principles of wound healing and wound management. In: R Bryant (ed.) *Acute and Chronic Wounds: nursing management.* Mosby Year Book, London.

12 Centre for Medical Education, University of Dundee (1992) *The Wounds Programme.* Centre for Medical Education, Dundee.

13 Baxter H (2004) Surgical wounds and their care. In: D Maxwell (ed.) *Surgical Techniques in Obstetrics and Gynaecology.* Churchill Livingstone, Edinburgh.

14 Martens M, Kolrud B, Faro S *et al.* (1995) Development of wound infection or separation after caesarean delivery: prospective evaluation of 2,431 cases. *J Reprod Med.* **40:** 171–5.

15 Bale S, Harding K and Leaper D (2000) *An Introduction to Wounds.* Emap Healthcare Ltd, London.

16 Bryant R (1992) *Acute and Chronic Wounds: nursing management.* Mosby Year Book, London.

17 Workman M (1995) Essential concepts of inflammation and immunity. *Crit Care Nurs Clin North Am.* **7:** 601–15.

18 Archer H (1990) A controlled model of moist wound healing. *J Exp Pathol.* **71:** 155–70.

19 Miller M and Collier M (undated) *Understanding Wounds.* Emap Healthcare Ltd, London.

20 Winter G (1962) Formation of the scab and the rate of epithelialisation of superficial wounds in the skin of the young domestic pig. *Nature.* **193:** 293–4.

21 Bryan J (2004) Moist wound healing: a concept that changed our practice. *J Wound Care.* **13:** 227–8.

22 Collier M (1996) Principles of optimum wound management. RCN Continuing Education Series. *Nurs Standard.* **17 July:** 47–52.

23 Lawrence J (1994) Dressings and wound infection. *Am J Surg.* **167:** S21–4.

24 Ovington L (1998) The well-dressed wound: an overview of dressing types. *Wounds.* **10 (Suppl. A):** 1–11A.

25 Russell L (2000) Understanding physiology of wound healing and how dressings help. *Br J Nurs.* **9:** 10–21.

26 Lock P (1998) The effect of temperature on mitotic activity at the edge of experimental wounds. In: A Lundgren and A Soner (eds) *Symposia on Wound Healing: plastic surgical and dermatologic aspects.* Molndal, Sweden.

27 Parker L (2000) Applying the principle of infection control to wound care. *Br J Nurs.* **9:** 394–404.

28 Gordon G and Lochhead D (1994) An outbreak of group A haemolytic streptococcus puerpal sepsis spread by the communal use of bidets. *Br J Obstet Gynaecol.* **101:** 447–8.

29 Williams C and Young T (1998) *Myth and Reality in Wound Care.* Quay Books, Salisbury.

30 Hampton S and Collins F (2003) *Tissue Viability.* Whurr Publications, London.

31 Barr J (1995) Principles of wound cleansing. *Ostomy/Wound Manag.* **41 (Suppl. 7A):** 15–21.

32 Pudner R (1997) Wound cleansing. *J Commun Nurs.* **11:** 30–6.

33 Enkin M, Keirse J, Neilson J *et al.* (2000) *A Guide to Effective Care in Pregnancy and Childbirth* (3e). Oxford University Press, Oxford.

4

Nutrition and its role in healing

This chapter contains an overview of the role of various nutrients in pregnancy, in particular identifying the nutritional influences on efficient wound repair following delivery. Some other factors that contribute to becoming 'well nourished' are also mentioned, as obviously having the optimum health to be able to heal quickly would be the ideal situation. The influence of nutrition on healing is such a vast subject that this chapter can only hope to provide a brief summary. However, if midwives want to expand on these issues, or indeed explore other aspects of nutrition and childbirth, there are many valuable references at the end of this chapter.

Early motherhood almost inevitably involves poor sleeping patterns, inadequate nutrition and psychological stress. Ensuring that women have sufficient knowledge of nutrition to enable them not only to have a healthy pregnancy, but also to possess the resources to heal efficiently following the birth may go some way towards contributing to a reduction in postnatal complications.

A small study in the USA found that most women had inadequate nutritional knowledge and their diets did not meet all of the nutritional requirements of pregnancy.[1] This also seems to be the case in the UK.[2]

The postnatal period is a time when many women embark on diets − the majority of first-time mothers are surprised at the amount of weight that is retained immediately post delivery,[3] and are highly motivated to lose weight. Midwives need to ensure that these women are aware of what their body needs to accomplish, and that good nutrition is necessary both to heal and to maintain good health at a time of increased stress. Therefore fad diets and/or decreasing valuable nutrients at this time will not be beneficial.

The midwife is the first-line adviser on all pregnancy matters, and nutrition is frequently a subject that concerns women. It often seems that the midwife has decreasing amounts of time to spend with a woman, and a growing number of issues to discuss, but she has a clear role as a health educator to offer advice on nutrition. Many women do a great deal of preparation for the baby. However, perhaps they should also be preparing themselves from a health perspective for the rigours of motherhood. By conveying this in a short-term way with definite objectives, midwives may be helping to optimise the woman's (and baby's) health with perhaps beneficial long-term effects. Nutritional advice and support can be seen not only as fulfilling the midwifery role as health promoter, but also as preconception care for the next pregnancy. There is also a knock-on effect on the rest of the family, as the mother is usually influential in the feeding of others.

Unfortunately, though, nutritional assessment and advice are not a routine part of midwives' care in the UK. Traditionally nutrition has not been emphasised in the midwifery curriculum, and current staffing levels may make it difficult for a midwife to include this subject comprehensively in her practice. Yet this subject may have more impact on a woman's health during pregnancy, and therefore on her health and that of the baby following birth, than almost any other intervention. However, in other parts of the world, nutritional teaching for the woman may play a much larger part in midwifery care.

Almost all studies on nutrition and pregnancy use two easy-to-measure criteria, namely the weight gain of the woman and the birth weight of the baby. Maternal weight gain in pregnancy is often seen as a 'test' of the well-being of the pregnancy. However, only the increase in the pregnant woman's lean body mass has a direct relationship to the baby's birth weight. All experienced midwives will have seen women who gained 'appropriate' or even excess weight and delivered a small newborn, and conversely women who gained little or no weight and whose baby was large. Because of these anomalies, it is no longer usual practice to routinely weigh women who begin pregnancy with a normal weight in order to assess fetal growth.[4]

A woman may also gain weight during pregnancy – whether a 'satis-factory' amount or in excess – but this is no guarantee that she is taking in a good diet with the nutrients that will help to protect her from infection and ensure efficient healing in the postnatal period.

Good nutrition for the woman will obviously benefit the fetus and newborn, but the specific needs of the mother should also be considered. There should perhaps be more emphasis on nutrition to provide optimum health for the woman, especially in preparing for and coping with labour and the postnatal period. Nutrient deficiency in pregnancy may not impact on the fetus, but may deplete the woman's stores so that she is prone to delayed healing and infection following the birth. Paying attention to the nutritional status of the woman could help to protect her from beginning motherhood in a compromised state.

I have told my husband many times that I had my dinner before he came in, so there should be plenty to go round for the children and himself. (1915)[5]

Malnutrition certainly played a part in the high level of maternal mortality and morbidity in the early 1900s in the UK. Today, in far too many parts of the world, many women who die of complications in childbirth might have survived if they had had sufficient nutritional resources.[6]

In Britain, historically the emphasis was on getting enough food. However, at present in the western world, the quality of food and the growing trends in obesity are the two areas on which attention is focused.[7]

Obesity is of particular concern in pregnancy, and the *Confidential Enquiries into Maternal Deaths*[8] have identified a strong relationship between obesity and complications around the time of childbirth. Assessment needs to be made either before or early in pregnancy, by means of measurements of body mass index (BMI), to ensure that women who are at potential risk receive the appropriate care.

Box 4.1 Calculation of BMI (body mass index)

Weight in kilograms divided by the square of height in metres $=$ BMI.

Underweight:	$<18.5 \, kg/m^2$
Normal:	$18.5–24.9 \, kg/m^2$
Overweight:	$25.0–29.9 \, kg/m^2$
Moderately obese:	$30.0–34.9 \, kg/m^2$
Obese:	$35.0–40.0 \, kg/m^2$
Severely obese:	$>40 \, kg/m^2$

Food guides, first devised in the USA in 1916, have been depicted as pyramids or parts of a circle suggesting what made up a good diet, although recommendations have changed many times over the years. One of the many changes that have occurred in the recommendations is the belief that if macronutrients were consumed in adequate quantities, micronutrients would also be included. However, some authorities believe that this may only be true when most food is close to its natural state.[7] Nevertheless, written information and guidelines are a useful back-up for midwives, and there are leaflets available that may be valuable for the woman who is planning pregnancy (the ideal time to implement these suggestions) or who is newly pregnant.

Physiology

A specified daily amount of each nutrient is necessary, which varies according to the individual and their circumstances. It must be possible to obtain this amount from the daily diet or from the body's stores of that nutrient. If it is obtained from stores, these will need to be replaced or they will become depleted, which can result in a deficiency state. However, it is difficult to determine what is an exact deficiency level of each nutrient, as many have no recognised criteria for clinical deficiency, especially in pregnancy. Even if clear-cut deficiency levels were identified, it would be more useful to aim for adequate intake and stores to ensure the ability to cope with times of decreased input or stress, and since these would be highly individualised, it seems that establishing general criteria would be of limited use. It must also be remembered that pregnancy enhances the absorption of many nutrients, so any criteria would need to reflect this.

Box 4.2   Three measures of nutritional status[7]

- *Anthropometric indicators* are measurements such as BMI, skinfold thickness and waist/hip ratio, which are compared with the general population for assessment.
- *Biochemical indicators*, such as levels of nutrients or their by-products, can be measured by some blood and urine tests (and hair tests, although not proven).
- *Clinical indicators* include changes in external appearances and actions. Many external signs can provide hints of deficiencies. For example, skin, hair and nails can show distinctive changes.

Many companies offer nutritional analysis services, and these are of variable usefulness. For example, hair analysis by post could obviously give rise to many misinterpretations, whereas if it was offered along with other tests by trained professionals, it might be valuable.

Influences on food intake

Physiological needs may have only a partial influence on what and how much is eaten. Food may be consumed without physical hunger – for instance, when a tempting food is available. Conversely food may not be consumed when hunger is present – for example, when distracted or dieting. Eating can meet psychological needs, and may relieve anxiety, boredom or depression. Food can also be seen as representing love or nurturing when it is related to parenting or feeding loved ones.

Food choices can be dependent on many factors other than knowledge of what is a 'healthy diet'. Choice may be limited by what is affordable or available. Food that was eaten as a child influences a person's choices as an adult. Some may avoid food which they feel was 'forced' on them, while other foods may be seen as a 'treat' or comfort food because of past experiences.

Many value judgements are attached to foods. For example, when eating alone people will often consume food that they would not eat in company. This may influence how a woman describes her diet to a midwife, and she may only include food that she perceives will be approved of by the midwife. Overall in the UK there has been a change in how we view food, and with the growing trend in obesity, many foods are seen as 'bad' and 'dangerous'.

In pregnancy and the puerperium, when perhaps a woman is only able to tolerate a small intake, or when time is very limited, concentration on nutrients is vital. Pregnancy is often a time when women report altered ability to taste certain foods, or 'morning sickness' may be present in a more extreme and prolonged manner, and this may also restrict their diet. A woman with a history of extreme dieting (or anorexia – see later in this chapter) may enter pregnancy with low reserves of many nutrients and thus be vulnerable.

The influence of culture must be considered, as many foods may be eaten or rejected due to traditional practices or religious beliefs. Most midwives in the UK will have cared for women whose family provides a traditional food specific for childbirth, recovering from birth or breastfeeding.

Changes in society

Allergies/intolerances

There appears to have been an increase in the prevalence of food allergies and intolerances over the past few decades. It has been suggested that this may be a result of increasing levels of pollutants entering the food chain, or the development of intensive farming practices. Alternatively, perhaps it is just that among an affluent society in a privileged position, identification of such allergies and intolerances is more likely.

Of particular interest to midwives is the increasing number of peanut allergies being reported (see later in this chapter).

Obesity

Suggested reasons for the rise in obesity in western societies include increased fat intake, perhaps contributed to by the trend towards eating outside the home. There have also been changes in society, such as irregular meal patterns, with 'mealtimes' no longer being seen as important, and easily accessible snacks being consumed whenever the need is felt. The decreasing levels of regular exercise taken are also seen as relevant.

Nutrient content of food

Changes in food technology (e.g. recently developed processing techniques such as irradiation or genetic engineering) may affect the nutrients in food, or the ability of the body to access those nutrients.[7]

Recommended diet

It is probably unrealistic to expect all women to follow a highly nutritious and balanced diet at all times. However, motivation with regard to optimising health has been noted to be extremely high during pregnancy. Furthermore, some women report an aversion to certain substances, such as coffee, when pregnant. This may have an organic basis in that the pregnant body is trying to ensure that only valuable substances enter the body.

Foodstuffs fall into four main categories, namely proteins, fats, carbohydrates and the micronutrients (vitamins and minerals) necessary for normal biochemical processes. Fibre, although not strictly a nutrient, also has an important role to play in a healthy diet.

Antioxidants are also vitally important. They protect the body by blocking the action of free radicals. Some free radicals are by-products of the natural destruction of bacteria, damaged cells and other waste products, but it seems increasingly likely that more are produced in response to increasing levels of pollution.[7] Free radicals can damage body cells and weaken defences against heart disease and cancer. The main antioxidants are vitamins C and E, selenium, zinc and beta-carotene. Midwives will be aware of the promising research on the possible effect of antioxidants on pre-eclampsia.[9]

Box 4.3   Energy content of foodstuffs

1 gram of carbohydrate	16 kilojoules (3.75 calories)
1 gram of fat	37 kilojoules (9 calories)
1 gram of protein	17 kilojoules (4 calories)
1 gram of alcohol	29 kilojoules (7 calories)

Proteins

Amino acids are the building blocks of proteins and are vital for structure and function. Most amino acids are derived from plants, and protein is obtained either by eating plants, or by eating animals that have eaten plants. Animal protein has a similar balance of amino acids to human protein. However, in vegetable protein the balance varies, so it is necessary to eat a wide range in order to obtain a good balance. The protein is utilised by breaking it down into amino acids and restructuring them according to need.

Each cell in the body contains protein both as part of its cell membrane and within its cytoplasm. Protein has a major role in the function of the immune system, as it is needed for normal cell division to produce cellular components. Antibodies and other vital agents are also composed of amino acids. Therefore protein deficiency will result in a defective immune system. Amino acids are necessary for the cell synthesis and division that are so vital for wound healing. A lack of protein leads to a decrease in angiogenesis, reduced proliferation of fibroblasts and endothelial cells, and reduced collagen synthesis and remodelling. It has been suggested that egg and milk proteins are particularly important for tissue repair after damage.[7]

Protein requirements are about 0.75 g protein/kg/day, and some authorities recommend slightly higher values. For example, the Department of Health[10] states that more than 1.5 g/kg/day would be excessive, but there is no clear evidence for this,[7] although it is suggested that extra high protein supplements may lead to fetal compromise or damage.[11]

The commonest sources of protein are meat, milk, bread, cereal, eggs, dairy products, fish, legumes, nuts and seeds.

Fat

Fat is a concentrated source of energy (37 kJ/g or 9 cal/g). Of all the macronutrients fat contains the most energy. More than twice as much energy is provided per gram of stored fat than per gram of carbohydrate or protein.

Animals use or store the fat that they ingest, or alternatively they can synthesise most fat from surplus energy that is consumed as carbohydrate or protein. Some plants contain fat (e.g. olives, nuts). The absorption of fat-soluble vitamins from the digestive tract depends on the presence and absorption of fats. Therefore individuals on very-low-fat diets may be at risk of deficiency of these vitamins.

Fatty acids

Most fatty acids can be produced by the body, but two cannot, namely *linoleic acid* and *linolenic acid*. Since both of these are necessary for health, they are known as essential fatty acids[12] and must be supplied by the diet. During pregnancy, especially in the early stages, the rapid growth of the fetus can lead to a decline in maternal essential fatty acid status.[13] Deficiency of these essential fatty acids can cause a recognised deficiency syndrome.

Polyunsaturated fats contain essential fatty acids which are necessary for normal brain development and for the production of some of the hormones that are needed for a healthy pregnancy.[14] They are also involved in the immune system response, and essential fatty acids in cell membranes contribute to stability through their role in helping to regulate metabolism. Fats and free fatty acids on the skin surface contribute to its waterproof properties and may be bactericidal.[7]

Fats can be subdivided into the following categories:

- *saturated* (e.g. animal fat, butter, cream, hard cheese, coconut oil, chocolate)
- *monosaturated* (e.g. vegetable oil, olive oil, meat, fish, avocado, eggs, peanuts)
- *polyunsaturated* (e.g. soya, sunflower oil, oily fish, nuts, seeds).

About 35% of energy intake is obtained from fats, but it is recommended that less than 10% should be obtained from saturated fat, to reduce the risk of heart disease.[12] It is recommended that 2–5 g of essential fatty acids should be consumed daily. Oily fish are a good source of polyunsaturated fatty acids, but because of possible contamination it is recommended that no more than two portions should be consumed per week.[14]

Carbohydrates

Carbohydrates are organic compounds that contain oxygen, hydrogen and carbon and are found in plants and animals. Their main function is to supply energy, and they should probably provide 50–55% of the energy required. Carbohydrates are subdivided into simple carbohydrates (monosaccharides, such as glucose, and disaccharides, such as sucrose) and complex carbohydrates (polysaccharides, such as starch).

Although glucose is the main carbohydrate in the body, it represents only a small proportion of dietary carbohydrate intake, as other carbohydrates are broken down into glucose (as well as other substances). There are some reserves of carbohydrate (glycogen) in the liver and muscles, but most excess carbohydrate intake is stored as fat. Carbohydrate metabolism changes during pregnancy, to promote the laying down of fat, and later to help to keep glucose levels higher for longer, so that the fetus can benefit.[15]

Carbohydrates supply energy, which is necessary for all body functions. Glucose is essential for the functioning of a number of organs, including the brain. Simple carbohydrates are found in fruits, honey, vegetables and milk. Complex carbohydrates are found in grains, vegetables, fruits and legumes.

Box 4.4　Fibre

Dietary fibre is a non-starch polysaccharide ('indigestible carbohydrate') derived from plant foods. It is believed to have a beneficial effect on many western diseases, such as heart disease, diabetes and gastric conditions. However, probably due to a lack of agreement about what exactly constitutes 'dietary fibre', there is no clear evidence for this, although a high-fibre diet is still regarded as a healthy option. Foods that are rich in dietary fibre are recommended during pregnancy to prevent constipation, which could lead to reduced appetite and thus decreased nutrient intake, as well as compromising the absorption of nutrients.

Vitamins and minerals (micronutrients)

Our understanding of vitamins and minerals is still incomplete, but they are known to be necessary for many of the chemical reactions that take place within cells. Vitamins, although necessary, are only needed in varying and usually small amounts, and in some cases vitamin overdoses can be fatal. The body has only a limited ability to store vitamins, so regular intake of some vitamins is necessary. Vitamins are present in animal and plant foods and can also be chemically synthesised in a laboratory.

Vitamin A (retinol)

Vitamin A is a fat-soluble vitamin that is stored in the liver. It has a role in red blood cell formation, so mild anaemia is often an early sign of deficiency. It also has a role as an antioxidant against free radical reactions, and has a key role in immunity, especially T-lymphocyte function and antibody response to infection. In addition, it contributes to the mucus-secreting properties of epithelial cells.

Vitamin A deficiency is strongly associated with depressed immune function and increased morbidity and mortality.[16] Deficiency of this vitamin also leads to decreased collagen synthesis and affects epithelialisation.

As a result of the use of feed supplements over the last 20 years, the levels of vitamin A stored in animal livers have increased radically, and as increased levels of vitamin A have been shown to be teratogenic, the consumption of liver and liver products is not recommended during pregnancy.[17] Similarly, fish oil supplements are not recommended, and if a woman is taking vitamin pills she should avoid those containing retinol (carotene-derived vitamin A should not be harmful).[14] However, in some parts of the world vitamin A sources are very limited, and a study conducted in Nepal showed evidence of a beneficial effect of vitamin A supplementation in pregnancy for women who were presumably deficient in vitamin A.[18]

Vitamin A is found in eggs, butter, milk products, liver, fish oils, carrots, red peppers, dark green leafy vegetables, broccoli, apricots, peaches and mangoes. Cooking does not generally reduce vitamin A levels, and in fact makes vitamin A in carrots more accessible.[7]

Vitamin B

Vitamin B is a complex group of vitamins. It is water-soluble, and therefore any excess is excreted in urine. Storage of vitamin B is limited (except in the case of vitamin B_{12}), and it is more easily lost during food preparation.

It has been suggested that the vitamin B complex can combat stress, and therefore paying attention to the levels of this nutrient may be particularly beneficial for new mothers. Several of the B vitamins are necessary for collagen reactions and also for bacterial resistance.

Vitamin B_1 (thiamine)

Vitamin B_1 has a major role in several metabolic reactions, in particular the release of energy from glucose. A deficiency can affect the nervous system, but most diets contain small amounts of this vitamin, so the onset of deficiency would be slow.

Vitamin B_1 is found in cereals (mainly wholegrain cereals, but it is added to white flour and breakfast cereals). It is also present in beans, seeds and nuts, liver and (in small amounts) in potatoes and milk. Vitamin B_1 absorption may be inhibited by alcohol.

Vitamin B_2 (riboflavin)

Vitamin B_2 is necessary for metabolic activities, to release energy from food, and is associated with growth. Adolescents are at particular risk of deficiency because their need is greater and they may have a reduced intake of this vitamin. Symptoms of deficiency are non-specific, but include cracked lips, burning eyes and oily skin.

Research in the Netherlands found that Dutch women consumed little vitamin B_2, but that when intake of this vitamin was increased, they gave birth to larger and longer babies.[18]

Vitamin B_2 is found in milk products, meat (especially liver), eggs and (in small amounts) in tea and dark green vegetables.

Vitamin B_3 (niacin)

Niacin is involved in energy release. Deficiency of vitamin B_3 may result in pellagra (a disorder characterised by diarrhoea, dermatitis and dementia). Alcoholics are particularly susceptible to this deficiency.

Nicotinic acid (niacin) is found in meat (especially liver), fish, peanuts, cereals, vegetables (especially potatoes) and (in small amounts) in coffee and cocoa.

Pantothenic acid (B vitamin)

Pantothenic acid is necessary for the metabolism of all macronutrients. It is found in a wide range of foods, including wholegrain cereals, meat, fish and poultry. Deficiencies do not normally occur because it is so readily available.

Biotin (B vitamin)

Biotin is also necessary for the metabolism of all macronutrients. As well as being widely available in many foods (especially liver, kidney, peanut butter, eggs and yeast), it can be synthesised by bacteria in the colon. Antibiotics can reduce the number of these bacteria, but since only a small amount of biotin is necessary, deficiency is very rare.

Vitamin B_6 (pyridoxine)

Vitamin B_6 is involved in many biological reactions, especially those associated with amino acid metabolism. A deficiency may be due to poor eating patterns, especially at times of increased demand, such as during pregnancy. Signs of deficiency may include anaemia, cracked lips or pellagra, and can be seen if the general diet is poor (e.g. in alcoholics).

Vitamin B_6 is found specifically in liver, wholegrain cereals, meat (including poultry), peanuts, walnuts, bananas and salmon. It is found in varying amounts in all animal and plant tissue.

Vitamin B_{12} (cobalamin)

Vitamin B_{12} is a good example of the co-dependence of nutrients. For example, it is necessary for folate use and for the metabolism of some fatty acids, and excess vitamin C can convert vitamin B_{12} into an inactive form. Vitamin B_{12} is also needed for the production of new cells.

A deficiency of this vitamin may result in the myelin coating of the nerve fibres becoming damaged. However, unless stores are low, vitamin B_{12} deficiency takes a long time to develop. An intrinsic factor is needed for absorption of this vitamin, and most cases of deficiency are due to lack of this factor (pernicious anaemia).

It has been noted in animal studies that nitrous oxide can compromise vitamin B_{12} metabolism, and there is a possibility (as yet uninvestigated) that a relationship may exist between the use of inhalation analgesia (entonox) in labour and anaemia resulting in fatigue postnatally.[19]

Vitamin B_{12} is found only in animal foods – that is, meat (especially liver), fish and milk. Vegans will need supplements or vitamin-enriched foods (e.g. some cereals) in order to obtain sufficient levels of vitamin B_{12}, and they are usually aware of this.

Folate (folic acid)

Folic acid deficiency affects rapidly dividing cells, particularly red blood cells and the cells that line the gastrointestinal tract. A deficiency may also affect white cell division, thereby influencing the effectiveness of the immune system. Folic acid is needed for the synthesis of nucleic acids (including DNA) and amino acids, and is therefore vital for new tissue formation.

Alcoholics usually have a decreased intake of folate, and alcohol also inhibits its absorption. Absorption by smokers may also be poor and they may require more folate.[7]

Pregnant women need to increase their intake of folic acid for their own health (20–25% of pregnant women may show signs of megaloblastic changes in bone marrow). Folic acid supplements are now routinely recommended for women to take prior to conception and in the first 12 weeks of pregnancy to reduce the incidence of neural-tube defects (NTD). Women who have had a previous pregnancy complicated by NTD are advised to take an increased folate supplement.[20]

Folate is found in green leafy vegetables (and in lesser amounts in other vegetables), liver, yeast, orange juice, whole wheat, tinned baked beans and fortified cereal and bread. Zinc can aid its absorption. However, folic acid is particularly susceptible to prolonged heating or re-heating, and all folate can be destroyed by cooking.

Vitamin C

Vitamin C is a water-soluble vitamin that aids the absorption of iron from non-meat sources. Although the protective aspect of vitamin C against scurvy is well known, this deficiency disease still occurs in the UK, in particular in teenagers who eat highly refined diets and among the homeless. Smokers are often deficient in vitamin C.

Vitamin C is essential for a healthy immune system and for efficient wound healing, and it is also an important antioxidant. It is essential for collagen synthesis, and a deficiency of this vitamin reduces tensile strength, impairs angiogenesis and increases capillary fragility.

Vitamin C is mainly found in vegetables and fruit. It is the least stable of all vitamins and can be easily destroyed by exposure to light and heat. Keeping vegetables hot after cooking continues the destruction of vitamin C, so there may be only a very minimal amount left after one hour.

Vitamin D

Vitamin D is a fat-soluble vitamin that maintains the serum calcium and phosphorus concentration necessary for functioning of nerves and muscles and supports their cellular processes. It can be synthesised by the body via the skin on exposure to sunlight. Dietary sources include butter, eggs, milk, meat and oily fish, and supplements are added to many manufactured foods (e.g. cereals).

Deficiency causes rickets in children and osteomalacia in adults. Individuals at risk include women who are largely housebound, particularly those who wear dense body-covering clothing (ultraviolet light can penetrate light clothing) and whose diet does not include dairy products and other dietary sources of vitamin D.

Vitamin K

Vitamin K is a fat-soluble vitamin that is needed for the normal binding of calcium in the bone matrix. It is necessary for blood clotting and is synthesised by bacteria, including those in the human gut. Vitamin K levels can therefore be compromised by antibiotics that destroy the normal gut bacteria.

Dietary sources of vitamin K are primarily plant foods such as green leafy vegetables (e.g. broccoli, cabbage, spinach) and peas, as well as liver and (in smaller amounts) other meat, dairy products and tea.

Vitamin E

Vitamin E is important for maintaining healthy skin and blood vessels, and therefore it is vital after birth for the repair of tissues. It may be the most important antioxidant vitamin, essential against free radical damage, and it works in conjunction with other nutrients, especially vitamin C. Deficiency is rare, but women who are exposed to a high free radical load (e.g. those who smoke, work in polluted environments or eat high levels of saturated fats) are at risk of having decreased levels.[7]

Vitamin E is found in vegetable oils, the germ of whole cereals, some green leafy vegetables, fruit, nuts, eggs and avocados.

Minerals

Most known minerals are believed to be essential, but it is worth noting that specific detailed knowledge of many minerals is still lacking, and the properties and roles of many minerals are as yet undiscovered. Only those minerals that have a known role in wound healing will be described.

The major mineral nutrients are calcium, phosphorus, potassium, sulphur, sodium, chloride and magnesium. The important trace minerals are iron, zinc, manganese, copper, iodide, chromium, cobalt and selenium.

When considering the intake of minerals it is most important to bear in mind that some minerals can interfere with the absorption of other minerals, usually by competing for the same carrier mechanism in the digestive tract. An example would be a large intake of calcium interfering with the absorption of iron and magnesium, or increased levels of zinc reducing the absorption of iron and copper. Furthermore, the efficiency of absorption of various minerals changes according to the body's needs. If the intake is high the absorption rate may drop, and if the need is greater (e.g. in pregnancy), absorption may be increased. Individual mineral supplements can therefore cause an imbalance of other minerals in the body.

Toxic minerals are harmful as they are usually difficult to excrete. A particular problem arises when they are similar to essential minerals and can therefore easily displace them. For example, strontium and caesium could replace calcium in bones and milk.

Many of the enzymes that are necessary for normal wound repair are derived from trace minerals such as copper, iron and zinc.

Calcium

Although calcium is vital for many of the body's functions, its specific role in healing is in blood clotting. About 30% of calcium intake is absorbed, although if the intake is high this percentage drops. During pregnancy and lactation, when the need for calcium is greater, the efficiency of absorption is increased.

Calcium is found in dairy products, sardines, canned salmon, baked beans and broccoli.

Copper

Copper is involved in the response to infection and is needed for the formation of collagen and elastin.

It is found predominantly in plant foods, the amount that is present being dependent on soil conditions.

Iron

There is evidence in western countries that an estimated 20–30% of women of childbearing age have negligible iron stores, although iron-deficiency anaemia is present in only about 2–8% of these individuals.[7] However, if supplementation of iron is considered in normal circumstances, the whole diet should be examined as the iron deficiency may be an indicator of a generally inadequate diet that may be lacking in other nutrients. A supplement of one nutrient may therefore result in unbalanced intake.

Iron is vital for the functioning of the immune system. Iron deficiency can decrease the oxygen-carrying capacity of blood, and anaemia may reduce healing due to decreased oxygen levels. Collagen synthesis is also dependent on iron.

Iron is found in red meat, dried fruit, leafy green vegetables and fortified cereals. Iron absorption is enhanced by taking it with vitamin C, and is reduced by taking it with wholegrain cereals, tea, coffee, nuts, chocolate, egg yolks, calcium and zinc (tea can reduce absorption by up to 60%).[7] The efficiency of iron absorption in pregnancy is increased (probably by about five- to ninefold).

Zinc

Zinc is vital for the immune system. It is particularly important in wound healing, as decreased zinc levels can inhibit epithelialisation and fibroblast proliferation and increase susceptibility to infection. As stress increases zinc uptake,[7] it is likely that a new mother will be accessing the necessary amount provided that her diet contains adequate levels of this mineral.

The results of animal studies suggest that there may be adverse effects in a pregnancy if zinc stores are deficient.[21] Where zinc deficiency has been identified in populations in the developing world, supplementation has not been shown to improve the outcome of pregnancy, although there is some limited evidence that it does improve the infant's immune function.[22] However, it must be remembered that there is always a risk that supplementation of one mineral will compromise the uptake of others.

Since zinc is removed by food processing, poor zinc status may become an increasing problem in the future.[7]

Magnesium

Magnesium has an important role in enzyme reactions and blood clotting, and it plays a vital part in the immune system. If the intake of calcium is high, absorption of magnesium may be restricted. Alcoholism reduces the amount of magnesium present.

Magnesium can be found in green leafy vegetables, whole grains and legumes. It is also present in hard water.

Individuals at risk of depleted nutrient stores

Box 4.5   Individuals at risk of depleted nutrient stores

Women following dietary restrictions
Adolescents
Smokers
Women with:
   closely spaced pregnancies
   low BMI
   eating disorders
   high alcohol intake
Women who live in poverty
Women who are taking the oral contraceptive pill

Dietary restrictions

Vegetarians and vegans, and indeed anyone who follows a special diet involving restrictions, may be at risk of nutritional deficiency during pregnancy.

However, most of those who make a specific lifestyle choice with regard to diet will have sufficient knowledge to achieve a balanced intake of nutrients. There is no evidence that vegetarian or vegan diets are harmful in pregnancy, but additional supplementation may be recommended.[23] More detailed information can be found at www.vegansociety.com and www.vegsoc.org.uk.

There is evidence that protein deficiency can occur in hospital patients,[7] and although this has not been specifically studied in pregnant women, there is no reason why it should not occur in these women, with their increased needs and the distraction of either a worrying antenatal admission or a new baby. This demonstrates the importance of the midwife considering the woman's nutritional intake during a prolonged hospital admission.

Adolescents

Age has been found to be strongly and significantly associated with reduced intake of most nutrients, demonstrating the risk for teenage pregnancies and the need for nutritional advice that targets teenagers.[24]

Poverty

It has been estimated that 25% of babies in the UK are born to families living in poverty.[24] These are mothers who are potentially at risk of decreased nutrient stores, which will impact on the condition of both the mother and the child. Midwives need to ensure that all women who need information about benefits receive it. This may be an area in which many SureStart midwives[25] become involved as this government initiative expands.

Eating disorders

Although a full discussion of this important subject is beyond the remit of this chapter, it must be mentioned, as the conditions that fall under this heading are a relevant and growing challenge for midwives. A recent study suggested that in London the incidence of pregnant women with eating disorders may be as high as 1%,[26] but it is acknowledged that the majority of people with an eating disorder will not be known to their carers. Women with severe anorexia may be easily identified, and indeed they will probably not come under midwives' care due to their reduced fertility. However, women with only mild anorexia or bulimia may be within the normal weight range.[27]

There seems to be an increase in obstetric complications (e.g. breech, pre-eclampsia and instrumental or operative complications) in women with eating disorders, which are sometimes difficult to relate to low weight or reduced nutritional status. However, these will all contribute to an increased need for healing in the postnatal period, when reduced stores of nutrients and decreased nutrition may slow healing and/or increase infection rates.

The midwife, as the primary caregiver in pregnancy, may be the first to suspect or be told about an eating disorder. It is vital that referrals are made to the relevant experts for long-term support and care. However, the midwife should continue to play an important role as part of the multi-disciplinary team throughout the woman's pregnancy and puerperium. Effective care could prevent some of the complications associated with poor or reduced nutrition.

Further information on this complex and ever-changing subject can be obtained from the Easting Disorders Association (www.edauk.com).

Smokers

Research has demonstrated that pregnant women who are smokers have a lower intake of most micronutrients, although after adjusting for variables only vitamin C and carotenoid intake was reduced.[28] Since there is evidence from trials of elderly patients that vitamin C supplementation aids healing, perhaps other individuals, such as smokers or teenagers (especially if the pregnant woman falls into both categories), should be advised to supplement their diet with vitamin C, or at least to increase their dietary intake, as this vitamin is so vital for healing.

Nutritional supplements

One international review that did examine maternal morbidity and nutrition found that most interventions (e.g. supplements) required further trials.[29]

There is much controversy as to whether or not nutritional supplements should be recommended in pregnancy. Healthy women who have regularly eaten a balanced and good-quality diet prior to pregnancy probably do not need artificial supplements, with the exception of folic acid. However, even for these women some would argue that elements beyond our control (e.g. vegetables grown in nutrient-deficient soil, chemicals in the food chain, etc.) may have put them at nutritional risk. A woman who has started pregnancy with poor nutritional reserves, or who finds that pregnancy-related illness severely restricts what she can eat, may need a supplement. Midwives are not professional nutritionists, and if they are concerned about any individual woman, a referral to a dietitian is probably the safest and most effective option.

When talking to a woman who wishes to take nutritional supplements, it is important to ensure that she understands that some supplements should be avoided in pregnancy, and that by taking some unnecessary individual supplements she may be putting herself at risk of malabsorption of other micronutrients (e.g. unnecessary iron supplementation may reduce the absorption of zinc).

Intake of extra vitamin C (which cannot be effectively stored) around the time of childbirth may aid healing if a woman's diet is lacking in fresh fruit and vegetables at this stage – which is very likely if she needs to eat hospital food for any length of time, and also in view of the lack of time available during the initial days of caring for a new baby.

What not to eat

Any infection can compromise healing, if only by reducing the woman's nutrient intake and stores. However, some infections directly relating to food can have an increased detrimental effect not only on the woman and her ability to heal, but also on the pregnancy and the fetus. Some foods have been identified for which there is clear evidence that a risk is involved in their consumption during pregnancy. Many other foods are subject to 'food scares', and there may not be such clear evidence of potential harm. However, women have the right to make up their own minds about these matters, and midwives must keep their advice up to date in order to be an effective resource.

Peanut allergy

There seems to be clear evidence of the risk of fetal exposure, or exposure through breast milk, to peanuts leading to a peanut allergy in the young child.[30] Since peanuts are added extensively to much of our food, there is a suggestion that over-exposure could have caused this increase in sensitivity.[31] Many women choose to avoid peanuts as far as possible both during pregnancy and while breastfeeding in order to reduce this risk.

Salmonella

The main symptoms of salmonella are diarrhoea and vomiting, perhaps accompanied by abdominal pain and fever. The woman may become very ill with this form of food poisoning, and her nutritional status will suffer. Raw or lightly cooked eggs have the potential to cause salmonella poisoning, and raw, rare or undercooked poultry or meat may carry salmonella and/or toxoplasmosis.

Listeria

Listeria may be asymptomatic or the woman may exhibit influenza-type symptoms. Several foodstuffs have the potential to carry listeria, including soft, unpasteurised or blue-veined cheeses, ready-to-eat cold poultry (which cannot be reheated), cooked–chilled convenience meals that are not heated through fully, ready-made salads and untreated milk.

Liver and liver products (e.g. pâté, liver sausage) have the potential to carry listeria and also contain increased levels of vitamin A, which has potentially teratogenic effects on the fetus.

Toxoplasmosis

Although the danger of toxoplasmosis being transmitted via cat faeces is widely known, it is not commonly known that many foods carry this risk as well. Raw, rare or undercooked poultry or meat, ready-made salads that have not been thoroughly washed, unwashed vegetables and goat's milk may all cause toxoplasmosis.

Food poisoning in general

Raw shellfish may carry a bacterium that causes food poisoning. Untreated milk may carry brucellosis or other bacteria and lead to food poisoning or listeria.

Conclusion

It is easy to become obsessed with individual nutrients and their presence in identified foods. However, it is worth bearing in mind that the more varied the diet, the more likely it is that it will contain all of the necessary nutrients. As Mary Barasi said in her valuable book, *Human Nutrition*:

> food which makes up a healthy diet is not very different from that which makes up a less healthy one ... it is proportions, cooking and preparation methods which may make the difference.[7]

It may be this message that is the most useful one for the midwife to convey to women in her care.

References

1 Fowles E (2002) Comparing pregnant women's nutritional knowledge to their actual dietary intake. *MCN Am J Matern Child Nurs.* **27:** 171–7.

2 Pearson S, Dimond H, Ford F *et al.* (1996) A survey of pre-pregnancy nutritional knowledge in family planning clinics. *Br J Fam Plann.* **22:** 92–4.

3 Stein A and Fairburn C (1996) Eating habits and attitudes in the postpartum period. *Psychosom Med.* **58:** 321–5.

4 Dawes M and Grudzinskas J (1991) Repeated measurement of maternal weight during pregnancy. Is this a useful practice? *Br J Obstet Gynaecol.* **98:** 189–94.

5 Davies ML (ed.) (1915) *Maternity: letters from working women.* Virago, London.

6 Harrison K and Bergstrom S (2001) Poverty, deprivation and unsafe motherhood. In: J Lawson, K Harrison and S Bergstrom (eds) *Maternity Care in Developing Countries.* RCOG Press, London.

7 Barasi M (1997) *Human Nutrition: a health perspective.* Arnold, London.

8 Lewis G (ed.) (2004) *Why Mothers Die: confidential enquiries into maternal deaths in the UK 2000–2002.* RCOG Press, London.

9 Chappell L, Seed P, Kelly F *et al.* (2002) Vitamin C and E supplementation in women at risk of pre-eclampsia is associated with changes in indices of oxidative stress and placental function. *Am J Obstet Gynecol.* **187:** 777–84.

10 Department of Health (1991) *Dietary Reference Values for Food Energy and Nutrients in the UK. Report of the Panel on Dietary Referency Values of the Committee on Medical Aspects of Food Policy.* Report on Health and Society Subject No. 41. HMSO, London.

11 Abrams B and Berman C (1993) Nutrition during pregnancy and lactation. *Prim Care.* **20:** 585–97.

12 Forsyth S and Hornstra G (2001) Essential fatty acids: maternal and infant nutrition. *Pract Midwife.* **4:** 34–6.

13 Al M, Houwellingen A, van Kester A *et al.* (1995) Maternal essential fatty acid patterns during normal pregnancy and their relationship to the neonatal essential fatty acid status. *Br J Nutr.* **75:** 55–68.

14 Hunter H and Dodds R (2003) *Food Facts for Pregnancy and Breastfeeding.* NCT Publications, Cambridge.

15 Blackburn T (2003) *Maternal, Fetal and Neonatal Physiology: a clinical perspective.* Saunders, St Louis, MO.

16 Azais-Braesco V and Pascal G (2000) Vitamin A in pregnancy: requirements and safety limits. *Am J Clin Nutr.* **71 (Suppl. 5):** S1325–33.

17 Dolk H *et al.* (1999) Dietary vitamin A and teratogenic risk: European Teratology Society discussion paper. *Eur J Obstet Gynecol Reprod Biol.* **83:** 32–6.

18 Christian P *et al.* (2000) Vitamin A or beta-carotene supplementation reduced symptoms of illness in pregnant and lactating Nepali women. *J Nutr.* **130:** 2675–82.

19 MacArthur C, Lewis M and Knox E (1991) *Health after Childbirth.* HMSO, London.

20 Medical Research Council Vitamin Study Group (1991) Prevention of neural tube defects: results of the Medical Research Council Vitamin Study. *Lancet.* **238:** 131–7.

21 Caulfield L *et al.* (1998) Potential contribution of maternal zinc supplementation during pregnancy to maternal and child survival. *Am J Clin Nutr.* **68 (Suppl. 1):** S499–508.

22 Shah D and Sachdev H (2001) Effect of gestational zinc deficiency on pregnancy outcomes: summary of observation studies and zinc supplementation trials. *Br J Nutr.* **85 (Suppl. 2):** S101–8.

23 Drake R, Reddy S and Davies J (1997) Are vegetarians receiving adequate dietary advice for pregnancy? *Br J Midwifery.* **5:** 28–32.

24 McLeish J (2002) 'All I ate was toast' – poverty and diet in pregnancy. *MIDIRS Midwifery Digest.* **12 (Suppl. 1):** S6–8.

25 Willyman-Bugter M and Tucker L (2004) Using Sure Start to develop an integrated model of postnatal midwifery care. *MIDIRS Midwifery Digest.* **14:** 379–82.

26 Turton P, Hughes P, Bolton H *et al.* (1999) Incidence and demographic correlates of eating disorder symptoms in a pregnant population. *Int J Eat Disord.* **26:** 448–52.

27 James D (2000) Easting disorders in pregnancy: challenges to nursing care. *Mother Baby J.* **5:** 37–41.

28 Mathews F, Ludkin P and Smith R (2000) Nutrient intakes during pregnancy: the influence of smoking status and age. *J Epidemiol Commun Health.* **54:** 17–23.

29 Tiran D (2003) European directives on nutritional supplements and herbal medicines: implications for midwifery practice. *MIDIRS Midwifery Digest.* **13:** 128–31.

30 Frank L, Maraian A, Visser M *et al.* (1999) Exposure to peanuts *in utero* and in infancy and the development of sensitization to peanut allergens in young children. *Pediatr Allergy Immunol.* **10:** 27–32.

31 Lack G, Fox D, Northstone K *et al.* (2003) Factors associated with the development of peanut allergy in childhood. *NEJM.* **348:** 977–85.

5
Perineal wounds

No matter how good the other outcomes may have been, most midwives will leave a birth in which the woman needed perineal sutures with a feeling of disappointment. This is an area where midwives often feel concerned about the trauma, and spend time reflecting on why the tear happened or why episiotomy was necessary, and whether there was any action that they could have taken to prevent it.

Unfortunately, maintaining up-to-date information and providing evidence-based practice in this area is not always easy, despite recent excellent publications (such as *Perineal Care: an international issue*, edited by Christine Henderson and Debra Bick[1]) devoted to the subject. However, much of the research available is limited, and women are also diverse in their perceptions and needs.

Attempts have been made to provide guidelines on how the midwife can best manage the second stage in order to avoid perineal trauma, but there are still no definitive answers. Some of the suggestions from the literature regarding different practices will be listed later in this chapter, because of course the ideal situation would be for a woman not to need healing of her perineum. However, current statistics show that about 75% of women with vaginal births will receive perineal sutures, and they will benefit from midwifery advice and care in order to achieve optimum perineal healing.

Episiotomy and tears

Although there are records of episiotomy being used for at least 200 years, in Britain midwives were historically proud of their ability to deliver a baby without trauma. One midwife who was trained in 1929 said '... and the whole thing that we were trained for was to protect the perineum, not to split it',[2] and another who was trained in 1935 stated that 'it was a disgrace to get a tear'.[2]

However, from around the 1950s to 1960s, coinciding with the movement of the majority of childbirth into hospitals, episiotomies were decreed necessary by obstetricians in charge for all primiparae and for anyone who had had a previous episiotomy[3] – in effect, for all women. This practice was widespread until it began to be questioned in the 1970s and research, especially that conducted largely by Jennifer Sleep and her colleagues,[4] showed that routine episiotomy offered no advantage to mother or baby, and in fact caused many potential complications for the woman. These findings are not only accepted today in the UK,[5] but have also been verified by international trials.[5,6] However, despite this body of work, routine or frequent episiotomy is often still performed in many countries around the world.[7]

Although its liberal use in the UK has diminished in recent years, in 1998 Garcia and colleagues[8] found that many episiotomies were still being performed for 'easier and quicker deliveries' or 'to avoid tears'. However, episiotomies are largely reserved for use with instrumental delivery, for cases of fetal distress where delivery needs to be expedited, or for the more controversial 'rigid' perineum, and are no longer recommended routinely.[5]

Nevertheless, many women sustain a spontaneous perineal tear, which may need suturing. Garcia et al.[8] found that of a total of 1951 spontaneous vaginal births, 57% of women had stitches (28% for an episiotomy and 29% for a tear), and other authors quote similar figures. Therefore care of these wounds is a common part of the postnatal care provided by all midwives.

Some research suggests that a tear will heal better than an episiotomy.[9,10] However, regardless of how it is sustained, perineal trauma with or without sutures will necessitate healing, and care and advice from the midwife may expedite this.

Perineal damage

Perineal damage is assessed as belonging to one of three or four categories.

- **First degree** – a tear which involves skin and subcutaneous tissue, with only a minimum amount or none of the muscle damaged. These tears are frequently left unsutured.
- **Second degree** – a tear which involves both skin and muscle layers (most commonly bulbocavernosus and superficial and deep transverse perineal muscles). An episiotomy will fall into this category, as both skin and muscle will be cut. When they occur spontaneously, it has been suggested that some second-degree tears may not require suturing (see later in this chapter).
- **Third degree** – a tear which involves the anal sphincter. This category may be subdivided according to how much of the sphincter is involved.[11]

- **Fourth degree** – a tear which involves the external and internal anal sphincter and mucosa. This category has traditionally been used more commonly in the USA, whereas in the UK any involvement of anal/rectal tissue has usually been classified as a third-degree tear. However, recommendations from the Royal College of Obstetricians and Gynaecologists now suggest that the above classifications should be used, while acknowledging that there is wide variation in interpretation of the terminology in practice.[12]

All third- and fourth-degree tears should be repaired in theatre with adequate regional or general anaesthesia to achieve relaxation of the sphincter.[12] There is a good argument that third- and fourth-degree tears, especially if complicated, should only be repaired by experienced professionals such as colorectal surgeons, and that the woman should be followed up until 12 months after the birth. Some maternity units have access to specialist colorectal nurses who may have a valuable part to play.

There is also evidence that not all third- and fourth-degree tears are correctly diagnosed at delivery,[13,14] although whether this is due to an attempt at denial by the carer or to the difficulty of the diagnosis is unclear.

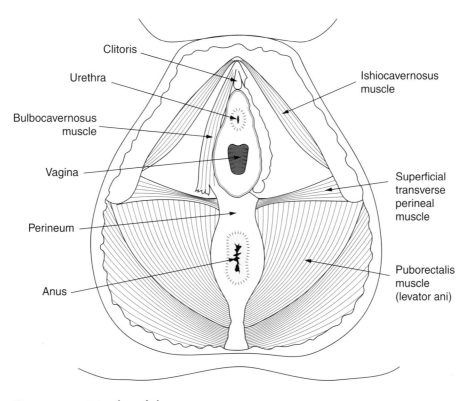

Figure 5.1 Muscles of the perineum.

Consequences of perineal trauma

Pain (short- and long-term) and dyspareunia

The importance of perineal care for the woman cannot be overstated. The vast majority of women suffer perineal pain[15] for at least the first few days following birth, and even those with intact perinea may report pain.[16,17] Although women expect pain during labour, postnatal pain usually comes as an unwelcome surprise, and can cause difficulty in undertaking infant care, interrupt bonding and potentially compromise the transition to motherhood.[18]

Pain can cause more than physical discomfort. The resulting reduction in mobility can lead to difficulty with breastfeeding and baby care, which can in turn make a new mother feel inadequate and lower her self-esteem, and this may lead to reduced self-care, especially lack of good nutrition, and result in a compromised immune system. Preoccupation with perineal problems has been reported to interfere with the development of a relationship with the baby,[17] and this may also make the woman feel less good about herself.

Even later in the puerperium when the midwife may consider the wound to be 'well healed' a woman may continue to feel pain. Glazener and colleagues,[19] along with many other researchers, found a substantial number of women reporting perineal pain for extended periods. In view of the fact that epithelialisation occurs long before the underlying structures have successfully remodelled (*see* Chapter 3), this is not surprising.

Long-term perineal pain and dyspareunia are not uncommon, and can affect up to 20% of women who have suffered trauma. A small Australian study by Abraham and colleagues[20] looked at how long it took women to feel comfortable in normal life following childbirth. These researchers studied a group of 93 women, of whom only four had had no perineal sutures. On average, perineal comfort when walking and sitting was not achieved until 1 month after childbirth, in 20% of women it took 2 months and in some it took as long as 6 months.

In the study by Abraham *et al.*,[20] it took 20% of the women more than 6 months to achieve comfort during sexual intercourse, and similarly dyspareunia was reported at 6 months by 31% of women in a study in the UK.[21] It is worth noting that dyspareunia can also affect women with intact perinea, and it is suggested that low oestrogen levels or other contributing factors not associated with perineal trauma may also be implicated.[22] However, regardless of the cause, the symptoms must be taken seriously. Dyspareunia, especially if ongoing, can seriously disrupt a woman's self-esteem and her relationship with her partner.[23]

There is obviously no doubt that perineal trauma has the potential for both short- and long-term effects, and can bring about such serious consequences as failure to breastfeed, disrupted maternal–infant attachment or relationship breakdown. Its importance cannot be over-emphasised.

Sleep

Pain may interfere with sleep, which also influences healing, and slower healing not only prolongs the pain but also predisposes to infection (*see* Chapters 2 and 3).

Urinary and faecal incontinence

A less common complication of perineal damage is urinary or faecal incontinence,[24,25] which can of course compromise a woman's physical and psychological well-being long into the future. It is suggested that 3–11% of women will report some form of faecal incontinence and around 19–30% will report urinary incontinence.[26] It is known that most morbidity is not reported to professionals,[25,27] so these figures can be regarded as conservative. Midwives must ask specifically about these symptoms, and then an appropriate referral can be made. Incontinence needs to be treated by professionals, and the Continence Foundation can provide expert advice and support (www.continence-foundation.org.uk or telephone helpline 0845 345 0165).

Although any trauma to the perineum has the potential for long-term continence complications, third- and fourth-degree tears have been most extensively studied in this context. Studies that show a lack of morbidity following third- or fourth-degree tears may not have considered all of the elements that are important to women. For example, Goldaber and colleagues[28] concluded that 'postpartum perineal morbidity after fourth-degree perineal repair is an uncommon event', after reviewing medical records and only looking at wound dehiscence, fistula formation and infection. Most women would also regard incontinence of faeces or flatus as significant morbidity, and this does not appear to have been addressed.

Faecal incontinence following childbirth was previously thought to be associated exclusively with third- and fourth-degree tears. However, it is now clear that for many women it is an unexpected consequence of uncomplicated childbirth. Although instrumental vaginal delivery was identified as an independent risk factor, it is worth noting that women who had had a Caesarean section (both emergency and elective) also complained of anal incontinence.[25] It is also extremely concerning that only 14% of the women who were identified in the research had sought medical advice for their symptoms.[25]

Occult damage to the anal sphincter has been identified by ultrasound examination in up to 44% of vaginal deliveries.[13,29] In follow-up assessments it has been demonstrated that up to 46% of women who had not been diagnosed with third- or fourth-degree tears, but who had newly occurring postnatal anal incontinence, still had symptoms 18 months later.[30] The impact of anal sphincter injuries in childbirth cannot be overestimated.

Risk factors for third- and fourth-degree tears have been identified as lack of manual perineal protection, a long second stage with pushing, no visualisation of the perineum,[31] instrumental delivery, midline episiotomy, infant birth weight and occipitoposterior (OP) position at delivery.[32]

There is no clear research to support the use of antibiotics and laxatives following repair of third- and fourth-degree tears, but this practice is recommended by the Royal College of Obstetricians and Gynaecologists guidelines[12] because of the importance of avoiding infection and wound dehiscence which could potentially compromise long-term function of the anal sphincter.

Labial lacerations

Many labial lacerations will be left unsutured, as they frequently do not bleed. However, consideration must be given to how the laceration will heal. If the anatomy will end up distorted, this may lead to dyspareunia and/or dissatisfaction of the woman due to compromise of her body image. There has even been a report of labial fusion, which necessitated surgical division, following an unsutured labial laceration.[33] A careful assessment of any labial trauma must be made in order to avoid serious consequences.

Emotional stress

Emotional stress may be increased by any adverse perineal event, leaving a woman with a vulnerable immune system, and thus hampering efficient healing, thereby creating a vicious circle.

For all of these reasons, if trauma does occur it is obviously best for the woman to heal as quickly and efficiently as possible, and the midwife needs to have a good understanding of the physiology of wound healing (see Chapter 3) and what actions can help or hinder this.

Suturing

Although there is evidence of perineal trauma being sutured during the 1800s when episiotomy was being widely discussed in the medical literature, a more normal treatment was to tie the woman's legs together for up to several weeks, until healing was complete.[34] However, especially following the movement of childbirth into hospital (and with the increase in routine episiotomy), suturing became more common and even routine. Historically doctors were responsible for all suturing (this often necessitated the admission to hospital of women who suffered perineal trauma during home birth), until suturing began to become a routine part of the midwife's role in the 1980s.

Suturing can obviously play a large part in the successful healing (and reduction of long-term sequelae) of perineal trauma.

Analgesia during suturing

Pain relief during suturing may not always be adequate. There is some evidence that pain experienced can be considerable and be a lasting memory of the birth experience.[35] In one study several women commented that the pain of stitching was worse than the pain of childbirth.[36] Since being sutured can never be a pleasant experience, with discomfort, embarrassment and exhaustion contributing to this, compounding the situation with inadequate analgesia will only cause more stress for the woman.

Second-degree tears

At present there is controversy in midwifery care as to whether or not all second-degree tears should be sutured. Some of the first research in the UK, in the early 1990s,[37] demonstrated that leaving selected second-degree tears unsutured led to as good or better outcomes in terms of speed of healing and the comfort of women.

More recent research[38] found poorer healing at 6 weeks in women who were not sutured. The authors of this randomised study regretted that so many women withdrew, and speculated that this may have been on the advice of under-confident midwives who wanted to avoid suturing. However, it may also be possible that some midwives advised suturing to those women who were randomised to the non-suturing group, because of 'jagged' or unaligned tears. Obviously even those who advocate non-suturing of second-degree tears will select individuals who will be not be sutured according to very careful criteria and not just the degree of tear. Another small randomised trial, which only considered 'minor' first- and second-degree tears, showed no difference in healing but an increased negative effect on breastfeeding in the sutured group.[39] It is likely that this will continue to be an area where the midwife's judgement will be of paramount importance.

Type of suture material

The type of suture material that is used may also influence the healing of the perineum. Absorbable synthetic suture material – polyglycolic acid (Dexon) and polyalactin (Vicryl) sutures – have been shown to reduce short-term pain, wound complications and dyspareunia compared with catgut.[40] However, the length of time that it takes synthetic sutures to be absorbed is a common complication, and this can cause discomfort or irritation. Removal of a suture that is too tight or is causing irritation often provides relief, and this should be done aseptically with sterile stitch scissors.[41]

Suturing technique

The method of suturing that is used by the midwife may have an influence on the degree of pain and the rate of healing. Overtight sutures can lead to necrosis and weaker wounds.[42]

A review of research comparing continuous subcuticular with interrupted suturing for perineal skin closure demonstrated less short-term pain when a subcuticular stitch was used.[43]

An attempt to make sutured perineal wounds more comfortable for the woman has led to experimentation with suturing only the inner layers and leaving the skin unsutured.[44] A study of 1730 women found a decreased incidence of long-term pain and dyspareunia in women with an unsutured skin layer.[45]

Timing of suturing

If suturing is necessary it should be done as soon as possible. When Garcia and colleagues[8] studied the experiences of women who needed stitches, they found that although 47% of cases were sutured immediately, 14% waited for 20–60 minutes and 8% waited for more than 60 minutes. Clearly it is difficult to draw exact conclusions from a purely statistical analysis (perhaps some of the women who had to wait had more urgent needs to be dealt with, such as a relaxed uterus or the baby requiring resuscitation), but the potential for even a small increase in blood loss, which may compromise the woman's ability to heal efficiently, should lead to every midwife aiming to have suturing completed as a matter of urgency. There may also be a psychological benefit to not delaying suturing, as the wait may produce increased anxiety in the woman and prevent her from focusing on the baby.[36]

Perineal wound dehiscence

The breakdown of a sutured perineum is always a cause for distress. The commonest reason is infection, and the commonest treatment has usually been antibiotic therapy and leaving the wound to heal by secondary intention (*see* Chapter 3). However, there is evidence that early re-suturing of the wound can lead to a good outcome,[46,47] although this may require further research, especially with regard to evaluation of the management of these wounds prior to re-suturing.

Postnatal midwifery care issues

The Royal College of Midwives' guidelines, *Midwifery Practice in the Postnatal Period*,[48] identify the fact that midwives have previously received limited evidence-based guidance on many aspects of midwifery care. There have recently been moves to rectify this situation by providing clear evidence for midwives to use in their practice. *Postnatal Care: Evidence and Guidelines for Management*[32] is one recent valuable resource that assesses long-standing routine care issues.

Historically women have been expected to remain in bed following childbirth for varying lengths of time. In the early 1900s in Britain women stayed in bed for 10–14 days,[2,49] and if in hospital they lay flat for the first 3 days. The midwife, either in hospital or when visiting at home, was responsible for the woman's hygiene, and 'vulval swabbing' at regular intervals during the day for up to 10 days was routine procedure, and various solutions were used for this.[50]

Today the assessment of the perineum is part of a midwife's normal postnatal check, whether by discussion with the woman or by physical examination. Midwifery care of the perineum is focused on preventing or treating pain and/or infection. Midwives (and the women they care for) are often surprised how quickly and successfully a perineal wound can heal. There is no doubt that the perineum is an ideal healing environment (*see* Chapter 3), as it is warm and moist with a good blood supply, so any interventions should not alter this.

Analgesia in the postnatal period

In the immediate postnatal period most women, including those with intact perinea, report some degree of perineal pain.[16,17,51] It is important that this pain is taken seriously and every attempt made to alleviate it.

A pain-free woman will be able to mobilise more easily and hopefully avoid complications that could lead to infection. There is also evidence that ongoing pain (and lack of sleep, which commonly accompanies pain) can depress the immune system and so compromise healing (*see* Chapter 2).

The most frequent treatment for perineal pain is oral analgesia, and the most common analgesic given to new mothers is paracetamol.[52] This is usually an effective treatment,[17] but there is some evidence that non-steroidal anti-inflammatory drugs (NSAIDs) are more effective.[51] Diclofenac suppositories in particular are often used prophylactically following suturing.[53]

There is some evidence that if women self-administer their drugs they are more satisfied with the pain management.[54]

Midwifery attitudes may in themselves have an analgesic effect. This is worth considering when analysing the effectiveness of any analgesia, especially when the research is quoted by those with a product to sell. If women are divided into two groups for research purposes, with one group being given treatment, the very fact of receiving treatment, especially by a sympathetic practitioner, may compromise the results.

As Jennifer Sleep wrote, 'The quality of personal individualised postpartum care is likely to be a major influence in reducing perineal pain and speeding recovery'.[52]

Comfort measures

Various comfort measures are in common use and are recommended either by midwives or by non-professionals. Some of these may not be ideal when considered from a strict 'wound-healing' perspective, but this aspect needs to be balanced against the advantage of the woman feeling comfortable.

Warm water/bathing

Water has always been widely used for therapeutic purposes,[55] and a warm bath can be very comforting holistically, as well as reducing perineal pain. There is some evidence that cold sitz baths (baths in which only the hips and buttocks are immersed) may be even more effective as an analgesic,[56] but they are not very appealing and also they do not fulfil the criterion of a constant temperature for optimum wound healing. Sitz baths have been studied in the USA and were not found to improve wound healing.[57] Immersion in warm water also changes the wound temperature, so this finding is not surprising, but the value of water as an analgesic, as well as contributing to basic hygiene requirements, must be considered.

Cold therapy

Ice packs and other versions of cold therapy are commonly used for local pain relief. A recent trial has reported that a chilled gel pack specifically designed for perineal application may be more beneficial than ice packs.[58] However, although the anecdotal evidence for pain relief by the use of ice or cold substances seems clear, a recent review of controlled trials did not support this.[59] Any cold application should lead to vasoconstriction, reduced oedema and therefore reduced pain. However, because restriction of blood flow can interfere with wound healing, cold therapy needs to be used with caution, perhaps only for short intervals and maybe not after 24–48 hours. Care also needs to be taken to prevent the cold pack from causing 'ice burns' on healthy tissue.

Herbal substances

Various herbal substances have been used as perineal 'soaks' on pads or as bath additives, but there is no clear evidence that these either reduce pain or improve healing. However, herbs such as comfrey leaf, lavender flower and calendula flowers,[60] made into a 'tea' and used as a perineal soak, have been reported to be effective, and descriptions of similar treatments are frequently found in advice columns in magazines for new mothers.

Herbal remedies should be prescribed by a qualified herbalist (a member of the National Institute of Medical Herbalists), and midwives should only give advice in areas where they are proficient.

Local pharmacological therapies

Anaesthetics (e.g. lignocaine) can be administered as a gel, spray or foam, and there is evidence that they can be effective in reducing pain.[52] Other preparations which contain steroids (e.g. Epifoam) have not been demonstrated to be effective,[61,62] and as steroids are known to compromise wound healing, the increased incidence of wound breakdown associated with the use of such preparations is not surprising.

Ultrasound and pulsed electromagnetic therapy

The use of ultrasound and pulsed electromagnetic therapy to treat perineal pain and trauma has been assessed, but the results of trials are inconclusive and further research is needed,[63] although when explored further these therapies may be of value.[64]

Pelvic floor exercises

It has been suggested that pelvic floor exercises can not only prevent or treat urinary incontinence,[65,66] but may also help healing, perhaps due to the increased blood supply. These exercises have also been reported to reduce pain,[67] perhaps by keeping the area flexible.

Other common suggestions

Some therapies that are aimed at achieving 'dryness' (e.g. the use of hairdryers on a cool setting or exposure to a heat lamp) can inhibit healing,[15] and clearly go against advice for achieving an optimum wound-healing environment.

It is possible that rubber rings, which have been used in the past to take the pressure off the perineum and thus increase comfort when sitting, may be harmful due to the potential for increased oedema caused by compression, which could in theory lead to increased pain and a reduction in healing. There is no evidence that they provide pain relief.[52] The Valley cushion, which was developed by a midwife, may prove to be an effective alternative.[68]

Possible midwifery influences in reducing perineal trauma

Antenatal

Nutritional advice to mothers

A detailed discussion of this topic can be found in Chapter 4.

Antenatal perineal massage

There is some evidence that antenatal perineal massage will reduce perineal trauma,[69,70] particularly in women aged over 30 years[71] and in those who have not had a previous vaginal delivery.[72]

Pelvic floor exercises

It has been suggested that if pelvic floor exercises are taught during the antenatal period, perineal trauma can be reduced.[73]

Intrapartum

As Sara Wickham wrote:

> *There is probably no one 'magic' way of assisting a woman to give birth that will ensure no perineal trauma, and in fact it may be that 'masterly inactivity' rather than activity may be the most appropriate 'action' to take.*[74]

However, every midwife should have enough knowledge of the different ways of assisting the birth process to enable her to help each woman in the way that is right for her as a unique individual.

Continuity of carer

This may contribute to reduced perineal trauma.[34] In a study of the effects of delivery by a known midwife,[75,76] those women who were delivered by a midwife who worked as a 'one-to-one' or 'caseload' midwife (who cared for them throughout their pregnancy) were found to have a reduced episiotomy rate, shorter labour and a decreased instrumental delivery rate. Therefore, not surprisingly, they experienced less perineal trauma. Studies have also shown that continuous intrapartum support in labour led to a decrease in the use of analgesia and decreased operative delivery rates, and therefore presumably better perineal outcomes.[77]

Avoiding epidurals

An epidural may lead to an increased likelihood of instrumental delivery (with associated episiotomy).[78] It has also been suggested that a prolonged second stage with epidural analgesia (even without instrumental delivery) may lead to an increase in the number of third-degree tears.[79] Caseload care by a midwife has been shown to reduce the epidural rate.[76]

Position during the second stage

Research findings are not consistent.[6] As there is no clear evidence as to which is the 'best' position, it may be that the woman's choice and her ability to change position according to how she feels may be the most important factors.[80–82]

Warm perineal compresses during the second stage

There is some evidence in the literature that warm perineal compresses may reduce perineal trauma,[83] perhaps by providing an analgesic effect.[84]

Perineal massage during the second stage

This is often debated by midwives who have different views. One line of reasoning is that massage during the second stage helps the perineum to stretch effectively, while according to the opposite theory handling of the perineum causes oedema and therefore increased risk of trauma. A randomised controlled trial[85] concluded that perineal massage causes no overall benefit or harm, which leaves midwives free to perform the procedure if they believe that it will help the individual concerned. Albers and colleagues[83] believe that the use of oils increases trauma.

Avoiding directed pushing

Although there is some suggestion that perineal outcomes are better with spontaneous pushing,[86] a meta-analysis of the available trials comparing sustained breath-holding pushing (Valsalva) with spontaneous pushing was inconclusive.[6] However, if 'slow and gentle' delivery (see below) protects the perineum, it would seem that violent pushing would be best avoided.

Slow and gentle delivery

This has been shown to be associated with an increase in the number of cases of intact perinea.[6]

Manual perineal protection and/or pressure to flex the fetal head during delivery

A large randomised trial (the 'HOOP' trial)[87] comparing hands on or hands poised (hands off) demonstrated a similar incidence of perineal trauma. However, there was slightly less perineal pain on day 10 in the 'hands on' group. There is some evidence that the lack of both 'manual perineal protection'[31] and 'manual help to the baby's head'[88] may result in an increase in third- and fourth-degree tears. Albers and colleagues[83] also state that control of the head may reduce perineal trauma.

References

1 Henderson C and Bick D (2005) *Perineal Care: an international issue.* Quay Books Division, MA Healthcare Ltd, Salisbury.

2 Leap N and Hunter B (1993) *The Midwife's Tale: an oral history from handywoman to professional midwife.* Scarlet Press, London.

3 Cronk M (1990) Midwives: a practitioner's view from within the NHS. *Midwives Health Visit Commun Nurs.* **26:** 58–63.

4 Sleep J, Grant A, Garcia J *et al.* (1984) West Berkshire perineal management trial. *BMJ.* **189:** 587–90.

5 Carroli G and Belizan J (2003) *Episiotomy for Vaginal Birth (Cochrane Review). The Cochrane Library. Issue 2.* Update Software, Oxford.

6 Renfrew M, Hannah W, Albers L *et al.* (1998) Practices that minimize trauma to the genital tract in childbirth: a systematic review of the literature. *Birth.* **25:** 1443–59.

7 Graham I and Davies C (2005) Episiotomy: the unkindest cut that persists. In: C Henderson and D Bick (eds) *Perineal Care: an international issue.* Quay Books Division, MA Healthcare Ltd, Salisbury.

8 Garcia J, Redshaw M, Fitzsimons B *et al.* (1998) *First-Class Delivery: a national survey of women's views of maternity care.* Audit Commission, London.

9 McGuiness M, Norr K and Nacion K (1991) Comparison between different perineal outcomes on tissue healing. *J Nurse Midwifery.* **36:** 192–8.

10 Larsson P, Platz-Christensen J, Bergman B *et al.* (1991) Advantage or disadvantage of episiotomy compared with spontaneous perineal laceration. *Gynecol Obstet Invest.* **31:** 213–16.

11 Keighley M, Radley S and Johanson R (2000) Consensus on prevention and management of postnatal obstructive bowel incontinence and third-degree tears. *Clin Risk.* **6:** 211–17.

12 Royal College of Obstetricians and Gynaecologists (2001) *Management of Third- and Fourth-Degree Perineal Tears Following Vaginal Delivery.* Clinical Green Top Guidelines; www.rcog.org.uk/guidelines

13 Faltin D, Boulvain M, Irion O *et al.* (2000) Diagnosis of anal sphincter tears by postpartum endosonography to predict fecal incontinence. *Obstet Gynecol.* **95:** 643–7.

14 Andrews V, Thakar R and Sultan A (2004) *Are midwives adequately trained to identify anal sphincter injury?* In: International Continence Society UK Proceedings, 11th Annual Scientific Meeting: 34. 18–19 March 2004.

15 Glossop C (1996) Perineal care after childbirth. *Health Visitor.* **69:** 96–9.

16 Albers L, Garcia J, Renfrew M *et al.* (1999) Distribution of genital tract trauma in childbirth and related postnatal pain. *Birth.* **26:** 11–15.

17 Greenshields W and Hulme H (1993) *The Perineum in Childbirth: a survey of women's experiences and midwifery practices.* National Childbirth Trust, London.

18 Boyle M (2000) Postnatal pain. In: M Yerby (ed.) *Pain in Childbearing: key issues in management.* Bailliere Tindall, Edinburgh.

19 Glazener C, Abdulla M, Russell I et al. (1993) Postnatal care: a survey of patients' experiences. BMJ. **1:** 67–74.

20 Abraham S, Child A, Ferry J et al. (1990) Recovery after childbirth: a preliminary prospective study. Med J Aust. **152:** 9–12.

21 Barrett G, Pendry E, Peacock J et al. (2000) Women's sexual health after childbirth. Br J Obstet Gynaecol. **107:** 186–95.

22 Goetsch M (1999) Postpartum dyspareunia: an unexplored problem. J Reprod Med. **44:** 963–8.

23 Comport M (1990) Surviving Motherhood. Ashgrove Press, Bath.

24 Goffeng A, Andersch B, Andersson M et al. (1998) Objective methods cannot predict anal incontinence after primary repair of extensive anal tears. Acta Obstet Gynecol Scand. **77:** 439–43.

25 MacArthur C, Bick D and Keighley M (1997) Faecal incontinence after childbirth. Br J Obstet Gynaecol. **104:** 46–50.

26 Pregazzi R, Sartore A, Bortoli P et al. (2002) Immediate postpartum perineal examination as a predictor of puerperal pelvic floor dysfunction. Obstet Gynecol. **99:** 581–4.

27 Glazener C, Abdalla M, Stroud P et al. (1995) Postnatal maternal morbidity: extent, cause, prevention and treatment. Br J Obstet Gynaecol. **102:** 286–7.

28 Goldaber K, Wendel P, McIntire D et al. (1993) Postpartum perineal morbidity after fourth-degree perineal repair. Am J Obstet Gynecol. **168:** 489–93.

29 Sultan A, Kamm M, Hudson C et al. (1993) Anal sphincter disruption during vaginal delivery. NEJM. **329:** 1905–11.

30 Zetterstrom J, Lopez A, Holmstrom KB et al. (2003) Obstetric sphincter tears and anal incontinence: an obstetric follow-up study. Acta Obstet Gynecol Scand. **82:** 921–8.

31 Samuelsson E, Ladfors L, Wennerholm U et al. (2000) Anal sphincter tears: prospective study of obstetric risk factors. Br J Obstet Gynaecol. **107:** 926–31.

32 Bick D (2005) Postpartum management of the perineum. In: C Henderson and D Bick (eds) Perineal Care: an international issue. Quay Books, MA Healthcare Ltd, Salisbury.

33 Arkin A and Chern-Hughes B (2002) Case report: labial fusion postpartum and clinical management of labial laceration. J Midwifery Women's Health. **47:** 290–2.

34 Graham I (1997) Episiotomy: challenging obstetric interventions. Blackwell Scientific Publications, Oxford.

35 Sanders J, Campbell R and Peters T (2002) Effectiveness of pain relief during suturing. Br J Obstet Gynaecol. **109:** 1066–8.

36 Green J, Coupland V and Kitzinger J (1998) *Great Expectations: a prospective study of women's expectations and experiences of childbirth.* Books for Midwives Press, Hale.

37 Head M (1993) *Non-suturing of tears to the perineum.* In: Proceedings of the International Confederation of Midwifery, 23rd International Congress, Vancouver, Canada: 809–22. 9–14 May 1993.

38 Fleming V, Hagen S and Niven C (2003) Does perineal suturing make a difference? The SUNS trial. *Br J Obstet Gynaecol.* **110:** 684–9.

39 Lundquist M *et al.* (2000) Is it necessary to suture all lacerations after a vaginal delivery? *Birth.* **27:** 79–85.

40 Kettle C and Johanson R (2003) *Absorbable Synthetic Versus Catgut Suture Material for Perineal Repair (Cochrane Review). The Cochrane Library. Issue 3.* Update Software, Oxford.

41 Bick D, MacArthur C, Knowles H *et al.* (2002) *Postnatal Care: evidence and guidelines for management.* Churchill Livingstone, Edinburgh.

42 Morrison M (1991) *A Colour Guide to the Nursing Management of Wounds.* Walfe Publishing, London.

43 Kettle C and Johanson R (2003) *Continuous Versus Interrupted Sutures for Perineal Repair (Cochrane Review). The Cochrane Library. Issue 3.* Update Software, Oxford.

44 Gordon B, Mackrodt C, Fern E *et al.* (1998) The Ipswich Childbirth Study. 1. A randomized evaluation of two-stage postpartum perineal repair leaving the skin unsutured. *Br J Obstet Gynaecol.* **105:** 435–40.

45 Grant A, Gordon B, Mackrodt C *et al.* (2001) The Ipswich Childbirth Study: one-year follow-up of alternative methods used in perineal repair. *Br J Obstet Gynaecol.* **108:** 34–40.

46 Ramin S, Ramun R, Little B *et al.* (1992) Early repair of episiotomy dehiscence associated with infection. *Am J Obstet Gynecol.* **167:** 1104–7.

47 Uygur D, Yesildaglar N, Kis S *et al.* (2004) Early repair of episiotomy dehiscence. *Aust NZ J Obstet Gynaecol.* **44:** 244–6.

48 Royal College of Midwives (2001) *Midwifery Practice in the Postnatal Period.* Royal College of Midwives, London.

49 Davies ML (ed.) (1915) *Maternity: letters from working women.* Virago, London.

50 Rhode M and Barger M (1990) Perineal care: then and now. *J Nurse Midwifery.* **35:** 220–30.

51 Dewan G, Glazener C and Tunstall M (1993) Postnatal pain: a neglected area. *Br J Midwifery.* **1:** 63–6.

52 Sleep J (1995) Postnatal care revisited. In: J Alexander, V Levy and S Roch (eds) *Aspects of Midwifery Practice: a research-based approach.* Macmillan Press, Basingstoke.

53 Searles J and Pring D (1998) Effective analgesia following perineal injury during childbirth: a placebo-controlled trial of prophylactic rectal diclofenac. *Br J Obstet Gynaecol.* **105:** 627–31.

54 Moffat H, Lavender T and Walkinshaw S (2001) Comparing administration of paracetamol for perineal pain. *Br J Midwifery.* **9:** 690–4.

55 Sleep J and Grant A (1988) Relief of perineal pain following childbirth: a survey of midwifery practice. *Midwifery.* **4:** 118–22.

56 Rambler D and Roberts J (1986) A comparison of cold and warm sitz baths for relief of postpartum perineal pain. *J Obstet Gynecol Neonatal Nurs.* **15:** 471–4.

57 Oladokun A (2000) A sitz bath does not improve wound healing after an elective episiotomy. *J Obstet Gynecol.* **20:** 277–9.

58 Steen M and Marchant P (2001) Alleviating perineal trauma – the APT study. *RCM Midwives J.* **4:** 256–9.

59 Hay-Smith E and Reed M (1997) Physical agents for perineal pain following childbirth: a review of systematic reviews. *Phys Ther Rev.* **2:** 115–21.

60 Lewis L (1994) Tea time: using herbs to help heal the unsutured perineum. *MIDIRS Midwifery Digest.* **4:** 455–6.

61 Greer I and Cameron A (1984) Topical pramoxine and hydrocortisone foam vs placebo in symptoms and wound healing. *Scott Med J.* **29:** 104–6.

62 Moore W and James K (1989) A random trial of three topical analgesic agents in the treatment of episiotomy pain following instrumental vaginal delivery. *J Obstet Gynaecol.* **10:** 25–39.

63 Hay-Smith E (1999) Therapeutic ultrasound for postpartum perineal pain and dyspareunia. *J Assoc Chart Physiother Women's Health.* **85:** 7–11.

64 Bibby P, Carrier, Davis N et al. (2000) A questionnaire reviewing current trends in the use of pulsed electromagnetic energy for the treatment of perineal trauma following vaginal delivery. *J Assoc Chart Physiother Women's Health.* **87:** 35–41.

65 Elia G and Bergman A (1993) Pelvic muscle exercises: when do they work? *Obstet Gynecol.* **81:** 283–6.

66 Glazener C, Herbison G, Wilson P et al. (2001) Conservative management of persistent postnatal urinary and faecal incontinence: a randomised controlled trial. *BMJ.* **323:** 593–6.

67 Sleep J and Grant A (1987) Pelvic floor exercise in postnatal care. *Midwifery.* **3:** 158–64.

68 Yearwood J (1991) The Valley cushion. *Midwives Chron.* **104:** 336.

69 Gomme C, Sheridan M and Brewley S (2003) Antenatal perineal massage. Part 1. *Br J Midwifery.* **11:** 707–11.

70 Gomme C, Sheridan M and Brewley S (2004) Antenatal perineal massage. Part 2. *Br J Midwifery.* **12:** 50–4.

71 Shipman M, Boniface D, Tefft M *et al.* (1997) Antenatal perineal massage and subsequent perineal outcomes: a randomised controlled trial. *Br J Obstet Gynaecol.* **104:** 787–91.

72 Labrecque M, Eason E, Marcoux S *et al.* (1999) Randomised controlled trial of prevention of perineal trauma by perineal massage during pregnancy. *Am J Obstet Gynecol.* **180:** 593–600.

73 Premkumar G (2005) Perineal trauma: reducing associated postnatal maternal morbidity. *RCM Midwives J.* **8:** 30–2.

74 Wickham S (2001) 'Perineal pampering' – before, during and after birth. *MIDIRS Midwifery Digest.* **11 (Suppl. 1):** S23–7.

75 Page L, Beake S, Vail A *et al.* (2001) Clinical outcomes of one-to-one midwifery practice. *Br J Midwifery.* **9:** 700–6.

76 Benjamin Y, Walsh D and Taub N (2001) A comparison of partnership caseload midwifery care with conventional team midwifery care: labour and birth outcomes. *Midwifery.* **17:** 234–40.

77 Hodnett E, Gates S, Hofneyr G *et al.* (2003) *Continuous Support for Women During Childbirth (Cochrane Review). The Cochrane Library. Issue 3.* Update Software, Oxford.

78 Lieberman E and O'Donoghue C (2002) Unintended effects of epidural analgesia during labour: a systematic review. *Am J Obstet Gynecol.* **186:** S30–68.

79 Donnelly V, Fynes M, Campbell D *et al.* (1998) Obstetric events leading to anal sphincter damage. *Obstet Gynecol.* **92:** 955–61.

80 Enkin M, Keirse M, Neilson J *et al.* (2000) *A Guide to Effective Care in Pregnancy and Birth* (3e). Oxford University Press, Oxford.

81 Gupta J and Hofmeyr G (2003) *Position in the Second Stage of Labour for Women Without Epidural Anaesthesia (Cochrane Review). The Cochrane Library. Issue 3.* Update Software, Oxford.

82 De Jonge A and Lagro-Janssen A (2004) Birthing positions: a qualitative study into the views of women about various birthing positions. *J Psychosom Obstet Gynecol.* **25:** 47–55.

83 Albers L, Anderson D, Cragin L *et al.* (1996) Factors related to perineal trauma in childbirth. *J Nurse Midwifery.* **41:** 269–76.

84 Page L (2000) *The New Midwifery: science and sensitivity in practice.* Churchill Livingstone, Edinburgh.

85 Stamp G, Kruzins G and Crowther C (2001) Perineal massage in labour and prevention of perineal trauma: randomised controlled trial. *BMJ.* **322:** 1277–80.

86 Chalk A (2004) Spontaneous versus directed pushing. *Br J Midwifery.* **12:** 626–30.

87 McCandlish R, Bowler U, Van Asten H *et al.* (1998) A randomised controlled trial of care of the perineum during the second stage of normal labour. *Br J Obstet Gynaecol.* **105:** 1262–72.

88 Pirharen J, Gronman S, Haadem K *et al.* (1998) Frequency of anal sphincter rupture at delivery in Sweden and Finland. *Acta Obstet Gynecol Scand.* **77:** 974–7.

6

Caesarean section wounds

Women were first reported to have survived a Caesarean section in the nineteenth century. Since then the rate of Caesarean section deliveries has increased dramatically, especially in the latter part of the twentieth century. The rising rates of Caesarean section delivery in the UK have recently been the focus of increased attention, and the numbers of Caesarean sections are also growing worldwide.[1] In the UK, rates have increased from 4% in the 1970s to 23% in 2003–04. Much publicity has been given to the suggestion that more women are requesting elective Caesarean sections, but in fact it is the emergency Caesarean section rate that has increased most rapidly. However, it has been suggested that if a woman requests an elective Caesarean section, 69% of consultants would agree to this,[2] although National Institute for Clinical Excellence (NICE) guidelines[3] have recently been produced to try to reverse this trend.

The varying rates of Caesarean sections in hospitals across the nation[4] may be thought to reflect local needs and perhaps pockets of deprivation, but in fact it is possible that the Caesarean section rates of individual hospital trusts may be more dependent on the maternity unit's culture than on external influences. It is also true that many factors other than maternal choice and hospital culture influence the rising rate of Caesarean sections, such as demographic and socio-economic considerations, and this debate is unlikely to be easily resolved.[1]

Meanwhile, as Caesarean sections have become more common, and of course much safer, an operative delivery – once a terrifying last resort for a pregnant woman – has certainly become more acceptable. Much of the improvement in maternal mortality and morbidity following Caesarean section has resulted from improved surgical and especially anaesthetic techniques. Before 1981 there were 30–50 anaesthetic deaths in the UK every three years, mostly related to general anaesthetics, while in 2000–02, only 6 deaths were recorded, none of which were attributed to regional anaesthesia.[5]

Clearly the safe use of blood transfusion and the widespread availability of antibiotics and intensive care units have also contributed to the improved outcome, and serious complications (*see* Box 6.1) or death are rare following Caesarean section today.

Box 6.1   Potential complications of Caesarean section

Haemorrhage
Pulmonary embolism or deep vein thrombosis
Infection (wound, endometritis, urinary tract infection)
Wound dehiscence/burst abdomen
Anaesthetic (general or regional anaesthetic accident)
Possible separation from baby (increased special care baby unit (SCBU) admissions)

(*see* Chapter 8 for details of endometritis and urinary tract infections)

Poor healing or non-healing of Caesarean section wounds is perceived to be a complication of the past. Nowadays women are more likely to concentrate their attention on the cosmetic aspects of the scar.[6] However, many women experience severe infection, wound breakdown, 'burst' abdomen, severe scarring, and occasionally the outcome is death.

Women's perceptions of the wound vary considerably. Many, especially those with no experience of previous surgical procedures, are surprised at the length of time for which they are aware of the wound or scar. The scar may feel numb for many months,[7] and there may be problems with the scarring itself (*see* Chapter 3).

The rate of wound infection following Caesarean section is very difficult to evaluate. Research has shown that only 47% of potential infection has occurred by day 7, with 78% occurring by day 14 and 90% by day 21.[8] After Caesarean section women are frequently discharged home from hospital on around day 4 or 5, and therefore it is unlikely that an infection will be diagnosed at this stage. Many infections will be suspected by the community midwife but diagnosed and treated by the GP, and many more infections will only be seen by the GP, as the community midwife will no longer be visiting. Therefore unless specific research is undertaken, the infection rate for Caesarean section by individual units (or indeed by individual surgeons) is impossible to evaluate.

Some studies have shown that infection rates may be as high as 25.3%,[9] but most Caesarean sections are by definition 'clean' surgery and should have an infection rate no higher than 2%.[10] More attention needs to be paid to this area, to ensure that women are not receiving sub-standard wound care nor, on the other hand, that they are being treated unnecessarily.

Wound care has changed, and continues to change rapidly, and the care of a difficult wound is outside the midwife's remit. Most hospitals will have expert nurse practitioners – tissue viability nurses or infection control nurses – with up-to-date expertise that the midwife can access when dealing with a difficult wound. If the woman is at home, community midwives often call upon district nurses, who also have relevant experience and expertise.

However, the midwife has a vital and multiple role in routine Caesarean section wound care. All midwives know that new mothers have a tendency to neglect their own physiological needs in favour of the needs of their infants, and therefore to begin with there is a role for education. Women need to know that the best way to care effectively for their new baby is by ensuring that their own health is optimal, and this involves attention to their own sleep and nutritional needs.

Box 6.2   Actions that may reduce the risk of infection

Education
Pain relief
Ensuring adequate nutrition
Ensuring good wound care practices
Identifying infections
Optimising the possibility of sleep in hospital
Reducing stress and increasing self-esteem

Actions which may prevent infection

Operation site preparation

It is known that if the operative site is shaved more than 12 hours pre-operatively there is an increased risk of infection.[11] Most women who are undergoing an emergency Caesarean section are unlikely to be able to take a pre-operative shower, and if the operation is due to failure to progress, they may have been relatively immobile in labour for many hours (with many different staff undertaking abdominal palpation). A wash with soap and water pre-operatively will remove most of the transient bacteria that have been acquired.[12]

Supporting the immune system

Good nutrition is vital for successful wound healing. Advice on optimising nutrition should be given routinely in the antenatal period, but if the woman's condition necessitates hospitalisation prior to Caesarean section, midwives may need to support and advise her with regard to her nutritional intake, especially if she is ill or anxious. There is evidence that even a short period of pre-operative fasting can significantly reduce nutrient levels,[13] and many women undergo emergency Caesarean sections after many hours in labour when food intake has been severely restricted or banned. Therefore it is extremely important for women to be aware that beginning labour with the best possible nutrient level would be advantageous.

If the woman is hospitalised prior to Caesarean section, it would be advantageous to encourage and enable as much good-quality sleep as possible. If antenatal ward space is limited, the midwife will have to be creative in order to meet the needs both of women in early labour, who may need to move around and make some noise, and of other women who need uninterrupted sleep. Following the operation, again midwives need to be aware that having as much sleep as possible will contribute to the woman's uneventful recovery.

Stress and anxiety levels can compromise the immune system (*see* Chapter 2) and wound healing (*see* Chapter 3), so midwives need to ensure that they do everything possible to make the woman feel relaxed and confident (e.g. by talking her through the information that she needs, or allowing flexible visiting by her partner).

Clinical issues

Caesarean section usually involves increased blood loss compared with a spontaneous vaginal delivery. It is not known exactly how much blood loss will be detrimental to an individual woman's condition, but it would be sensible to ensure that she is not anaemic either before or after the operation, as this may impair wound healing.

It has been demonstrated that although drains are not usually recommended, they may reduce the incidence of infection in obese women.[14]

In the UK, it is recommended that all women undergoing Caesarean section should receive intravenous antibiotic prophylaxis during surgery,[15] on the basis of clear evidence that this decreases the rate of post-operative endometritis and wound infection. However, the question arises as to why these mostly young healthy women undergoing 'clean' surgery are prone to infection. Perhaps giving greater attention to many of the issues raised in this book would change this situation.

Pain relief

Effective pain relief is necessary for optimal wound healing, as pain can compromise the immune system (*see* Chapter 2). Good pain control is also necessary, especially following hospital discharge, to allow good-quality sleep and to increase mobility. Decreased mobility can lead to a woman neglecting her own needs, especially concerning nutrition. However, increased ability to mobilise comfortably can also lead to more positive feelings, increased confidence with regard to childcare and increased self-esteem, all of which contribute to a healthy immune system.

All women will need analgesia following Caesarean section. There is evidence that perhaps carers may be unable to accurately assess women's level of pain,[16] and also hospital routines (e.g. regular drug rounds) may mean that women do not receive analgesia at the right time for them. Obviously the optimum delivery of analgesia would involve women themselves being in control of its administration, and research studies have shown that regimes which use patient-controlled analgesia (PCA) are most effective.[17] Being in control of their oral medication also seems to increase women's satisfaction with analgesia.[18]

The goal of analgesia after Caesarean section is to achieve good pain relief without sedation, in order to ensure maximum mobility.[19] Consideration must also be given to the transfer of narcotic drugs to breast milk.[20] The use of non-steroidal anti-inflammatory drugs (NSAIDs) such as diclofenac (Voltarol) can reduce the amount of opioid medication that is needed.[21]

There is also evidence that oral analgesia only can be successfully used after Caesarean section, and of those women who took part in a trial comparing oral morphine and oral dipyrone, all requested only 25% of the dosage allowed.[22] Certainly if effective pain relief could be achieved by using only tablets, this could potentially not only increase the woman's mobility and ability to care for her newborn by ridding her of the need for intravenous lines for PCA, but would also help her to feel more 'normal'.

Infection

Box 6.3   Features of wound infection

Spontaneous discharge of pus before or after suture removal
Opening of a wound
Non-purulent discharge containing pathogens such as coliform bacteria
  or *Staphylococcus aureus*
Spreading cellulitis

Most wound infection appears after 7 days (although group A and B beta-haemolytic streptococci may appear within 1–2 days). *Confidential Enquiries into Maternal Deaths in the UK*[23] found that the organism most commonly responsible for serious obstetric infection is beta-haemolytic streptococcus (Lancefield Group A – Lancefield Group C and G were less common). Lancefield Group B consists of normal vaginal flora, and is mainly a problem for the baby, although serious infection may also occur in the mother. Laboratory reports may not differentiate between Lancefield groups, but *Confidential Enquiries* suggests that this would be good practice.

It is difficult to diagnose mild infection in a Caesarean section wound, as many of the signs can be confused with normal wound healing (*see* Chapter 3). However, it is important to get it right in order to avoid unnecessary treatment with antibiotics, especially when the mother is breastfeeding, as these are transferred to the baby, which is a serious concern for many women.

Most signs and symptoms of a wound infection are an exaggeration of normal wound healing physiology. They include the following.

- **Erythema (redness).** This may be the normal inflammatory process, but it may progress to cellulitis.
- **Discharge.** A small amount of serous fluid may be normal, but large amounts or the presence of pus is not.
- **Pain or tenderness of the wound.** This may be normal (especially in a woman who is trying to care for her baby, with little sleep or nutrition, in the early postnatal period), but increasing pain, especially when resting, would be a worrying sign.
- **Oedema.** This may be part of the normal healing process, or even a local reaction to suture material, or it may be a sign of infection.
- **Pyrexia.** This may indicate a wound infection, or an infection elsewhere in the woman, or it may be associated with breastfeeding and engorgement.
- **Malaise.** This is a common postnatal and post-operative symptom, but it may also indicate that the woman is unwell.
- **Microbiology culture.** This can be positive, not only when infection is present, but also due to contamination or colonisation.

We live in harmony with the vast majority of the micro-organisms that are found within us. Many of these are commensals, but all can give rise to infection if conditions are favourable. An infectious agent often originates from the woman's own genital tract. This explains the increase in post-operative infection in women who labour prematurely, as a vaginal infection is often the cause of preterm labour. However, *Staphylococcus aureus* is the identified bacterium in about 25% of cases, and these are probably of environmental origin, not due to endometritis.[24]

Risk groups

Many studies have identified groups of women who are at increased risk of developing infection following a Caesarean section (*see* Chapter 3 for a more general list of women at risk of infection).

Box 6.4   Characteristics of women at risk of postnatal infection following Caesarean section

Increasing age
Obesity
Anaemia
Smoking
Premature labour
Prolonged labour (with increased number of interventions, especially vaginal examinations)
Prolonged rupture of membranes
Chorioamnionitis

Obesity has been shown to be a factor that increases the risk of developing a wound infection.[25] Although women who are obese may lack nutrients that are vital for healing, there also appears to be a relationship between infection/ wound breakdown and obesity. It has been suggested that this is due to a technically more difficult operative procedure, and the fact that blood vessels within fat are more easily torn.[26]

There is also evidence that higher infection rates occur in emergency rather than elective Caesarean sections.[27] However, in view of the fact that most emergency operations will be performed either following a long, debilitating labour, or as a result of an emergency such as haemorrhage – and whatever the reason, the likelihood is that the woman will be under extreme stress – this finding is not surprising.

Although childbearing women are not generally considered to be 'old', some research has demonstrated that there is an increased risk of infection following Caesarean section in women over 35 years of age.[28]

The most important risk factor for endometritis is Caesarean section,[29] but it must be borne in mind that pre-existing infection may be an underlying cause of preterm rupture of membranes or preterm labour (both of which increase the risk of Caesarean section being performed). Furthermore, many women who undergo Caesarean section will have had a prolonged labour, with an increased number of vaginal examinations and possible other interventions (e.g. internal fetal monitoring) which predispose to infection.

Good wound care

The principles of good wound care were discussed in Chapter 3, so only specific issues will be considered here.

The basis of maintaining a warm and moist environment is to keep the wound covered. Most dressings are removed after 24 hours, and research has demonstrated that in the case of a surgical wound this should not lead to any increase in infection.[30,31] However, further research is needed in these days of concern about hospital hygiene and MRSA (methicillin-resistant *Staphylococcus aureus*) and other multi-resistant organisms (*see* Chapter 8). Consideration should be given to the use of an appropriate film dressing (e.g. OpSite Post-Op), which would enable a woman to bathe or shower[32] and allow the wound to be visualised, while still providing protection against wound contamination.[33,34]

The disadvantages of routine wound cleaning were discussed in Chapter 3, but if necrotic tissue or excessive exudate is present, cleaning will be necessary. This should be done by irrigation, using a pre-packed single-use irrigation device, or a 35-ml syringe and a 19-gauge needle to obtain the ideal pressure. Wiping or swabbing the wound with gauze or other materials can traumatise the healthy or healing tissue.[11]

Nutrition

There has recently been a general move towards early feeding after Caesarean section. Evidence from a survey of UK maternity units showed that in most cases it is midwives who decide when women can start to eat and drink post-operatively, and the time period ranged from less than 1 hour to more than 24 hours after surgery.[35] A Cochrane Review[36] reported that there appears to be no reason to limit oral intake routinely following Caesarean section, although the trials that were reviewed defined 'early' feeding as 6–8 hours after surgery.

Avoiding hunger and thirst may improve women's well-being generally. A study in which women were given regular diets within 8 hours of surgery (that involved regional anaesthesia only) found that they had a shorter hospital stay.[37] Following Caesarean section under general anaesthesia, women who started oral intake after 4 hours and had their intravenous infusions discontinued at that time suffered no more complications than a control group, and showed earlier initiation of breastfeeding and earlier ambulation, as well as reporting increased satisfaction.[38]

One of the main worries for the midwife when initiating early – or indeed immediate – feeding of women after Caesarean section is the issue of paralytic ileus. The research evidence does not appear to support this concern,[39] although one study showed an increase in mild ileus symptoms in women whose Caesarean section operation lasted for longer than 40 minutes.[37] Since it is suggested that handling of the bowel may predispose to a paralytic ileus, it may be useful for the midwife who will be caring for the woman immediately post-operatively to be informed of the extent to which this occurred, and to adapt her care with regard to offering oral intake accordingly.

Less common complications

Haematoma

One large study showed a rate of 3.5% for haematoma following Caesarean section.[40] The consequences will of course depend on the severity of the bleed, but haematomas can contribute to anaemia and pain, and provide a good medium for infection.[41]

Wound breakdown and dehiscence

Wound breakdown and partial or total dehiscence 6–10 days post-operatively is usually associated with infection or poor wound healing in a compromised woman, or it may be due to a technical failure of surgery. It can be an emergency situation that requires prompt attention. Uterine scar dehiscence from a previous Caesarean section scar is seen in less than 2% of women during the next pregnancy, whether they have a trial of labour or routine repeat Caesarean section. Many of these cases are asymptomatic and of no clinical importance,[42] but those that occur in labour can compromise the health of both the mother and the baby, and necessitate an immediate Caesarean section. An *incisional hernia* post Caesarean section occurs when the deep layers of tissue dehisce but the superficial layers heal. Additional surgery will probably be required, but this is not usually an emergency.

Pressure area ulceration, necrotising fasciitis and antibiotic-resistant infection

See Chapter 8 for a discussion of these conditions.

References

1 Kennare R (2003) Why is the caesarean section rate rising? *MIDIRS Midwifery Digest.* **13**: 503–8.

2 Al-Mufti R, McCarthy A and Fisk N (1996) Obstetricians' personal choice and mode of delivery. *Lancet.* **347:** 544.

3 National Institute for Clinical Excellence (2004) *National Collaborating Centre for Women's and Children's Health Commissioned by the National Institute for Clinical Excellence (NICE). Caesarean section.* Royal College of Obstetricians and Gynaecologists, London.

4 Francome C, Savage W, Churchill H *et al.* (1993) *Caesarean Birth in Britain.* Middlesex University Press, London.

5 Lewis G (ed.) (2004) *Why Mothers Die: confidential enquiries into maternal deaths in the UK 2000–2002.* RCOG Press, London.

6 Jourdan T (2002) Scarred for life? Not these mums. *Daily Telegraph.* 22 July.

7 Chippington-Derrick D, Lowdon G and Barlow F (1996) *Caesarean Section: your questions answered.* National Childbirth Trust, London.

8 Weigelt J, Dryer D and Haley R (1992) The necessity and efficiency of wound surveillance after discharge. *Arch Surg.* **127:** 77–82.

9 Beattie P, Rings T, Hunter M *et al.* (1994) Risk factors for wound infection following caesarean section. *Aust NZ J Obstet Gynaecol.* **34:** 298–302.

10 Wilson J (1995) *Infection Control in Clinical Practice.* Bailliere Tindall, London.

11 Parker L (2000) Applying the principle of infection control to wound care. *Br J Nurs.* **9:** 394–404.

12 Babb J (2000) Decontamination of the environment, equipment and the skin. In: G Ayliffe, A Fraise, A Geddes *et al.* (eds) *Control of Hospital Infection* (4e). Arnold, London.

13 Goodson W, Jensen J, Gramja-Mena L *et al.* (1987) The influence of a brief preoperative illness on postoperative healing. *Ann Surg.* **205:** 250–5.

14 Allaire A, Fisch J and McMahon M (2000) Subcutaneous drain vs suture in obese women undergoing caesarean delivery: a prospective randomized trial. *J Reprod Med.* **45:** 327–31.

15 Smaill F and Hofmeyr G (2000) *Antibiotic Prophylaxis for Caesarean Section (Cochrane Review). The Cochrane Library. Issue 3.* Update Software, Oxford.

16 Olden A, Jordan E, Sakima N *et al.* (1995) Patients' vs nurses' assessment of pain and sedation after caesarean section. *J Obstet Gynecol Neonatal Nurs.* **24:** 137–41.

17 Rayburn W, Geranis B, Ramadei C *et al.* (1988) Patient-controlled analgesia for post-caesarean section pain. *Obstet Gynecol.* **72:** 136–9.

18 Moffat H, Lavender T and Walkinshaw S (2001) Comparing administration of paracetamol for perineal pain. *Br J Midwifery.* **9:** 690–4.

19 Boyle M (2000) Postnatal pain management. In: M Yerby (ed.) *Pain in Childbearing: key issues in management.* Bailliere Tindall, Edinburgh.

20 Ravin D (1995) Narcotic analgesics and breastfeeding. *J Hum Lactation.* **11:** 47–50.

21 Siddik S, Aouad M, Jalbout M *et al.* (2001) Diclofenac and/or propacetamol for postoperative pain management after caesarean delivery in patients receiving patient-controlled analgesia with morphine. *Reg Anesth Pain Med.* **26:** 310–15.

22 Jakobi P, Weiner Z, Solt I *et al.* (2000) Oral analgesia in the treatment of post-caesarean pain. *Eur J Obstet Gynecol Reprod Biol.* **93:** 61–4.

23 Lewis G (ed.) (2001) *Why Mothers Die: confidential enquiry into maternal deaths in the UK 1997–1999.* RCOG Press, London.

24 Owen J and Andrews W (1994) Wound complications after caesarean sections. *Clin Obstet Gynecol.* **37:** 842–55.

25 Rasmussen K, Linnet K, Jensen H *et al.* (1998) Morbidity after caesarean section in obese women. *Acta Obstet Gynecol Scand.* **77:** 782–3.

26 Martens M, Kolrud B, Faro S *et al.* (1995) Development of wound infection or separation after caesarean delivery: prospective evaluation of 2,431 cases. *J Reprod Med.* **40:** 171–5.

27 Allen V, O'Connell C, Liston R *et al.* (2003) Maternal morbidity associated with caesarean delivery without labor compared with spontaneous onset of labor at term. *Obstet Gynecol.* **102:** 477–82.

28 Magee K, Blanco J, Graham J *et al.* (1994) Endometritis after caesarean: the effect of age. *Am J Perinatol.* **11:** 24–6.

29 Bick D, MacArthur C, Knowles H *et al.* (2002) *Postnatal Care: evidence and guidelines for management.* Churchill Livingstone, Edinburgh.

30 Meers P, Jackson W and McPherson M (1994) *Hospital Infection Control for Nurses.* Chapman & Hall, New York.

31 Chrintz H, Vibits H, Cordtz T *et al.* (1989) Need for surgical wound dressing. *Br J Surg.* **76:** 204–5.

32 Bhattacharyya M, Bradley H, Holder S *et al.* (2005) A prospective clinical audit of patient dressing choice for postoperative arthroscopy wounds. *Wounds UK.* **1:** 30–4.

33 Boyle M (2001) Caesarean section wound management: a challenge for midwives. *Pract Midwife.* **4:** 20–3.

34 Ovington L (1998) The well-dressed wound: an overview of dressing types. *Wounds.* **10 (Suppl. A):** 1A–11A.

35 Worthington L *et al.* (1999) Attitudes to oral feeding following caesarean section. *Anaesthesia.* **54:** 292–6.

36 Mangesi L and Hofmeyr G (2002) *Early Compared With Delayed Oral Fluid and Food after Caesarean Section (Cochrane Review). The Cochrane Library. Issue 3.* Update Software, Oxford.

37 Patolia D *et al.* (2001) Early feeding after caesarean: randomized trial. *Obstet Gynecol.* **98**: 113–16.

38 Al-Takroni A *et al.* (1999) Early oral intake after caesarean section performed under GA. *J Obstet Gynaecol.* **19**: 34–7.

39 Kramer R *et al.* (1996) Postoperative management of caesarean patients: the effect of immediate feeling on the incidence of ileus. *Obstet Gynecol.* **88**: 29–32.

40 Van Ham M, van Dongen P and Mulder J (1997) Maternal consequences of caesarean section. A retrospective study of intra-operative and postoperative maternal complications of caesarean section during a 10-year period. *Eur J Obstet Gynecol Reprod Biol.* **74**: 1–6.

41 Gemer O *et al.* (1999) Sonographically diagnosed pelvic hematomas and post-cesarean febrile morbidity. *Int J Gynecol Obstet.* **65**: 7–9.

42 Enkin M *et al.* (2000) *Effective Care in Pregnancy and Childbirth.* Oxford University Press, Oxford.

7

Alternative healing and complementary therapies

This chapter will give a brief outline of some of the most common complementary therapies and any relevant research or opinions on their use in pregnancy and childbirth in relation to healing. Most of these therapies claim to produce a decrease in stress and anxiety, and this may have positive benefits in enhancing the immune system and healing (*see* Chapters 2 and 3). Any therapies that can deliver increased relaxation for a new mother will probably have definite positive effects in supporting an efficient immune system, as increased rest and sleep are of proven benefit.

The midwife may have a role as an alternative practitioner herself, and many midwives are augmenting their midwifery skills with qualifications in various complementary therapies. However, if she does not, her role is to encourage women to access qualified practitioners when they want to use these therapies, and perhaps to advise them on how to do this. The Complementary Maternity Forum has been set up in the UK for midwives who have an interest in complementary therapies, and it may be able to advise on local practitioners.

Midwives should also ensure that they are aware of various common therapies, as part of Rule 7 of the *Midwives' Rules and Standards* clearly states:

> *Homeopathic and herbal medicines are subject to the licensing provisions of the Medicines Act 1968. A number of these however have product licences but have not been evaluated for their efficacy, safety or quality, and you should look to the best available evidence to inform women. A woman has the right to use homeopathic and herbal medicines. However, if you believe that using the medicines might be counterproductive, you should discuss this with the woman.*[1]

In 1999, the Royal College of Midwives issued Position Paper 10a on *Complementary Therapy and Midwifery*.[2] It emphasised that midwives should 'never attempt to undertake any complementary therapy or give alternative forms of care for which they have not received formal recognised training'.

Midwives may also be bound by the terms of their employment. Discussion with managers must therefore be arranged by midwives before using complementary therapies in their practice.

However, midwifery and complementary therapies do seem to have a natural affinity, and midwives have been noted to be the professional group that is most likely to use complementary therapies.[3] One reason for this may be that the philosophy of midwifery, which puts the woman and her choices at the centre of care, is similar to that of most complementary therapies, where the emphasis is on holistic treatment. Indeed, the fact that there is a journal entitled *Complementary Therapies in Nursing and Midwifery* highlights the connection.

Examples of the involvement of midwives with complementary therapies are common. For instance, a complementary therapy clinic was set up in Northampton in 1999, and since then has not only increased the range of therapies that it offers, but has also been involved in the training of a growing number of midwives in a wide range of therapies.[4]

Pregnancy and the puerperium is a vulnerable time for many women. Choosing to use complementary therapies, because women need to make a conscious and deliberate choice to access them (whether from their local midwife or through a private practice), can be an empowering act that may thus have benefits over and above those of the therapy itself.

Touch

Many midwives will instinctively touch, stroke or hold the hand of a woman in distress or pain. Indeed, some women may spontaneously reach out for the midwife first at these times. Touch, such as palpating contractions during labour, can sometimes be seen more as communication, comfort or validation than as a clinical action.[5] One study has described women attributing their ability to cope during labour to touch – both by their partners and by their midwives.[6] It has also been noted that massage can facilitate communication,[7] adding psychological benefits to the physical ones.

The use of touch to promote well-being has been identified from the earliest recordable time, and was described in cave drawings and written documents from the Orient 5000 years ago.[8] However, there is a difference between therapeutic touch and casual touch for the purpose of stress reduction.

Therapeutic touch is a technique whereby the practitioner assesses and treats various areas of the body in order to rebalance and redirect energy, and is sometimes used in nursing care in North America.[8] In therapeutic touch, the hands of the practitioner are usually held above the skin, rather than in contact with it. The most important effects are considered to be inducing relaxation, reducing anxiety and pain, and promoting healing.[9]

Studies that have examined the use of touch, together with massage, during labour show that anxiety and pain can be reduced, thereby decreasing the levels of catecholamines,[10] which will make labour more efficient. It has also been demonstrated that massage therapy can reduce anxiety and stress hormones during pregnancy, which in one small study[11] decreased obstetric and postnatal complications, including premature labour. This study also noted that women reported better sleep. A reduction in anxiety and stress can improve the functioning of the immune system, and can thus make healing more efficient, so this may be particularly useful in the postnatal period.

Spiritual healing

Spiritual healing has also been referred to as faith, psychic, paranormal or mental healing. Spiritual healing is generally given as laying on of hands (with the hands lightly touching or near to the body), or it can be given from a distance with the healer sending healing mentally.[12]

Some research has been done on spiritual healing during pregnancy and labour, with reports that women feel labour has been 'eased' and that newborns seem to have received benefits as well.[12] There appears to be evidence for improvement of postoperative pain, healing of wounds and treatment of anxiety, the latter being a symptom that responds well to spiritual healing.[12]

Acupuncture

Acupuncture has been used in China since about 3000 BC, and it is part of traditional Chinese medicine. It involves the insertion of fine needles into specific points on the body, by which process acupuncture helps the body to correct itself by realigning or redirecting energy.[13]

Acupuncture is commonly used for physiological pain relief, and a study of symptoms such as back pain, symphysis pubis dysfunction and sciatica demonstrated increased well-being in the women who received this treatment.[14]

There are many studies that point to the efficacy of acupuncture in treating various types of infection through changes in the immune system.[15] There are also reports of its use for the induction of labour, and to provide analgesia during labour[15] – which, if successful, can improve the outcome for the woman by reducing the need for other interventions that may make increased demands on the immune system.

The practice of acupuncture often includes moxibustion, a related technique that involves the application of heat from the burning of the herb mugwort at the acupuncture points. For pregnant women, the commonest reason for using moxibustion is to turn a breech presentation to a cephalic one,[16] a procedure that is gaining acceptance in mainstream midwifery and obstetrics, and which may help to increase the normal birth rate, thus avoiding the need for a Caesarean section.

Aromatherapy

Aromatherapy is the use of essential oils extracted from plants to improve or maintain health and well-being. These oils can be administered by diffusion through the air, by inhalation, by absorption through the skin (with or without massage), or in a compress or mouth rinse, or in wound care. In the UK it is not usual to take these oils internally, but such a practice is adopted in France.[17]

Although essential oils are commonly regarded as a pleasant way to achieve a burst of energy or relaxation, it may be less well known that there are many reported toxic effects of various oils. This could be particularly important during pregnancy, when some oils may have teratogenic effects or even lead to a miscarriage. Aromatherapy practitioners will be aware of the safety aspects as well as the appropriate use of each oil.

There is some research evidence that aromatherapy can reduce the use of epidurals, thereby presumably reducing the need for other interventions.[18]

It has been demonstrated that aromatherapy can be successfully introduced into a maternity service by giving specific training to all midwives in a unit to work within identified guidelines and using a limited number of oils, to the benefit of the women and the satisfaction of the midwives.[19]

Many of the common oils have antiseptic, antibacterial, antiviral and/or antifungal properties, and may therefore be extremely useful in preventing infection or in general healing. Those oils that combat anxiety or promote relaxation and sleep will also be valuable in maintaining the strength of the immune system.

Homeopathy

Homeopathy was first described in the early 1800s, and has long been part of recognised care in the UK, being included as an officially approved method of treatment when the NHS was established,[20] and still being practised within the NHS today, albeit only in limited areas.

Homeopathy is the principle of 'treating like with like' and uses a greatly diluted – or 'infinitesimal' – dose of the remedy. In fact, the greater the dilution, the more potent the remedy is thought to be. Homeopathy is based on treating the 'whole person', and therefore all prescriptions are individual.

There have been reports of specific homeopathic remedies being valuable in reducing bruising and postnatal pain,[21] and these remedies are often used by women following birth. However, most homeopathic treatment is given not for specific ailments but to improve a person's general health, thereby enabling them to withstand disease, or to achieve maximum health for conception, pregnancy and childbirth. It is therefore not unusual for midwives to care for women who have been accessing homeopathy for some time, and have a range of remedies for any potential problems that may arise, as well as to bolster the immune system to combat the inevitable stress of childbirth and new parenthood. A woman may 'self-prescribe' to suit her particular symptoms. However, although the remedy will not be harmful, she will probably get a better result and avoid unwanted effects if she consults a professional homeopath.

Shiatsu

Modern shiatsu is based on a Japanese technique that uses massage and acupressure to balance the different energy flows within the body in order to promote a sense of well-being.[22] The purpose of the use of shiatsu in the context of healing is to reduce stress, which should promote a competent immune system. However, it may also have an effect on conditions during labour (e.g. induction, augmentation, pain relief or retained placenta),[23] which would reduce the need for other interventions and therefore benefit the woman.

Midwives are becoming increasingly involved in providing shiatsu, as there are short courses available specifically for midwives that provide training in skills directly related to their practice.

Reflexology

Reflexology is an ancient therapy that involves applying pressure to various defined reflex points (representing 'zones' of the body), most commonly on the foot, although they can also be on the hands or ears.

A feeling of well-being and relaxation is reported by most individuals who receive reflexology,[24] and this will of course be beneficial in supporting the immune system. However, there have also been reports of 'emotional' or 'tearful' reactions, and reflexology practitioners consider that this may be a 'healing crisis'.[25]

Other uses of reflexology mentioned in the literature as being of specific benefit to childbearing women include reduction of leg oedema[26] in pregnancy, and maintenance of lactation in stressful situations.[27] There is also some evidence that reflexology can play a part in alleviating 'normal' pregnancy-related nausea and vomiting,[28] which would certainly improve the woman's general well-being, as well as helping to maintain a good nutritional status.

References

1 Nursing and Midwifery Council (2004) *Midwives' Rules and Standards.* Nursing and Midwifery Council, London.

2 Royal College of Midwives (1999) *Position Paper 10a: complementary therapy and midwifery.* Royal College of Midwives, London; www.rcm.org.uk

3 NHS Confederation (1997) *Complementary Medicine in the NHS: managing the issues.* NHS Confederation, Birmingham.

4 Ager C and Gadsden W (2005) Complementary therapies: moving forward. *RCM Midwives J.* **8:** 224–5.

5 Boyle M (1992) *Midwifery influences on women's positions during childbirth.* Unpublished MSc dissertation, South Bank University, London.

6 Birch E (1986) The experience of touch during labour: post-partum perceptions of therapeutic value. *J Nurse Midwifery.* **31:** 270–6.

7 Tiran D (2001) Massage and aromatherapy. In: D Tiran and S Mack (eds) *Complementary Therapies for Pregnancy and Childbirth* (2e). Bailliere Tindall, Edinburgh.

8 Sayre-Adams J (2001) Therapeutic touch. In: D Rankin-Box (ed.) *The Nurse's Handbook of Complementary Therapies* (2e). Bailliere Tindall, Edinburgh in association with the Royal College of Nursing, London.

9 Fischer S and Johnson P (1999) Therapeutic touch: a viable link to midwifery practice. *J Nurse Midwifery.* **44:** 300–9.

10 Field T (2000) *Touch Therapy.* Churchill Livingstone, Edinburgh.

11 Field T, Hernandez-Reif M, Hart S *et al.* (1999) Pregnant women benefit from massage therapy. *J Psychosom Obstet Gynecol.* **20:** 31–8.

12 Benor D (2001) Spiritual healing research. In: D Rankin-Box (ed.) *The Nurse's Handbook of Complementary Therapies* (2e). Bailliere Tindall, Edinburgh in association with the Royal College of Nursing, London.

13 Downey S (2001) Acupuncture. In: D Rankin-Box (ed.) *The Nurse's Handbook of Complementary Therapies* (2e). Bailliere Tindall, Edinburgh in association with the Royal College of Nursing, London.

14 Hope-Allen N, Adams J, Sibbritt D *et al.* (2004) The use of acupuncture in maternity care: a pilot study evaluating the acupuncture service in an Australian antenatal clinic. *Compl Ther Nurs Midwifery.* **10:** 229–32.

15 Budd S (2000) Acupuncture. In: D Tiran and S Mack (eds) *Complementary Therapies for Pregnancy and Childbirth* (2e). Bailliere Tindall, Edinburgh.

16 Grabowska C (2005) The development of a study on 'turning the breech using moxibustion'. *MIDIRS Midwifery Digest.* **15 (Suppl. 1):** S32–4.

17 Stevensen C (2001) Aromatherapy. In: M Micozzi (ed.) *Fundamentals of Complementary and Alternative Medicine* (2e). Churchill Livingstone, Philadelphia, PA.

18 Burns E (2002) Aromatherapy in childbirth. *MIDIRS Midwifery Digest.* **12:** 349–53.

19 Jardin M (2002) Aromatherapy: introduction into a maternity service. *Pract Midwife.* **5:** 14–15.

20 Castro M (1993) *Homeopathy for Pregnancy, Birth and Your Baby's First Year.* St Martin's Press, New York.

21 Worden J (2003) Homeopathy in antenatal, perinatal and postnatal care. *MIDIRS Midwifery Digest.* **13:** 173–5.

22 Yates S (2005) Shiatsu and acupressure in practice. *MIDIRS Midwifery Digest.* **15 (Suppl. 1):** S35–8.

23 Yates S (2003) *Shiatsu for Midwives.* Books for Midwives Press, London.

24 Cull G (2002) *Reflexology and relaxation in a maternity hospital.* Proceedings of the International Confederation of Midwives. Midwives and Women Working Together for the Family of the World, Vienna. 14–18 April 2002.

25 Mackereth P (1999) An introduction to catharsis and the healing crisis in reflexology. *Compl Ther Nurs Midwifery.* **5:** 67–74.

26 Mollart L (2003) Single-blind trial addressing the differential effects of two reflexology techniques versus rest on ankle and foot oedema in late pregnancy. *Compl Ther Nurs Midwifery.* **9:** 203–8.

27 Tipping L and Mackereth P (2000) A concept analysis: the effect of reflexology on homeostasis to establish and maintain lactation. *Compl Ther Nurs Midwifery.* **6:** 189–98.

28 Tiran D (2004) *Nausea and Vomiting in Pregnancy: an integrated approach to care.* Churchill Livingstone, Edinburgh.

8

Common and rare areas of sepsis: midwifery issues

Both common and rare issues are covered in this chapter, but all of them are infections that are relevant to midwifery practice and are of course vitally important to the women who suffer from them.

Breast infections

Mastitis

Mastitis can affect many women following childbirth. The prevalence is unclear, but an Australian study suggests that it is about 20%.[1] Not only can mastitis cause pain and inconvenience for the woman, but also she may stop breast-feeding as a result of this condition, which could impact on the baby's health.

Symptoms of breast inflammation and pain, pyrexia, systemic aches and general malaise usually occur early in the postnatal period, and may last for 1 to 12 days.[2] The initial inflammation may be non-infective and caused by distension of the lactiferous ducts due to a blockage. Treatment at this stage is aimed at clearing the blockage, and increased feeding, a change in feeding position or hot compresses may all help to achieve this. However, if the condition does not resolve within 6 to 8 hours, the risk of infection or abscess formation is increased,[3] and the woman may need to commence antibiotic treatment.[4] In a study that investigated the experience of mastitis, it was reported that women found reducing their activity level was beneficial to their recovery,[5] a finding that is not surprising in view of the working of the immune system (*see* Chapter 2).

The presence of damaged nipples may predispose to infection by providing a means of entry,[6] and therefore midwifery support to prevent nipple trauma can be extremely beneficial.

Nipple trauma

Most nipple trauma is caused by incorrect positioning, and traditionally it has been believed that if the positioning is improved the trauma will heal spontaneously.[7] However, optimum wound care theories support the promotion of a moist warm environment, and the use of a suitable dressing,[8] or just ensuring that moisture is present by the use of expressed breast milk,[9] may speed healing.

Candidiasis

A less common form of breast infection is mammary candidiasis (thrush), which may cause the woman to stop breastfeeding due to the pain in her nipple and breast. Diagnosis can be made from the symptoms (flaky or shiny skin, painful nipples or pain in the breast) and from microbiology of the skin and milk specimens. Early treatment is important to enable the woman to continue breastfeeding.[10]

Urinary tract infections

A urinary tract infection is defined as a bacterial count higher than 100 000 ml in two successive clean catch specimens or a catheter specimen.[11]

Diagnosis of a urinary tract infection is often made on the basis of dipstick analysis ('bedside testing'), but research findings have shown that dipsticks should only be used as a screening tool. Although findings of protein/blood or leucocytes may indicate that a midstream specimen should be cultured, the most significant finding on a dipstick is a positive nitrates reading.[12]

Box 8.1   Possible symptoms of urinary tract infection

Haematuria
Frequency of micturition
Retention of urine
Lower abdominal or loin pain
Incontinence
Dysuria
Difficulty in voiding
Systemic symptoms (e.g. pyrexia, tachycardia)

Urinary tract infections may occur in around 5–10% of pregnant women,[13] and about 30% of these women may develop acute pyelonephritis if asymptomatic bacteriuria is left untreated.[14] Asymptomatic bacteriuria may also be associated with premature labour or low-birth-weight babies. In addition, it has been suggested that urinary tract infections may even have such far-reaching effects as increasing the risk of cerebral palsy in the baby,[15] but more research is needed to confirm this.

During the postnatal period the prevalence of urinary tract infections is around 2–4%.[16] Caesarean section is a major risk factor, along with a previous history and other variables that probably involve catheterisation (e.g. preeclampsia or eclampsia, placental abruption,[17] instrumental delivery and administration of an epidural[18]).

It may be beyond the means of midwives to reduce the conditions that lead to the risk of a urinary tract infection (although it could be argued that increased midwifery support may influence the epidural rate). However, the majority of catheterisation and care is provided by midwives, and this could be the area in which midwives can make a difference to the well-being of women. By scrupulously following good practice recommendations (*see* Chapter 9), not only may the woman be protected from developing an infection and requiring antibiotic treatment, but also she may avoid the need for activation of her immune system to fight invading bacteria (even if this is successful and no infection develops), which uses a considerable amount of her resources at a time when she needs to heal, produce breast milk and also cope with stressors such as reduced sleep and nutrient status.

It has been suggested that cranberry juice may be useful for the prevention and treatment of urinary tract infections, although there is no clear evidence for this.[19,20]

Pressure area injury

Increasing numbers of pressure sores are being identified in women following labour,[21] and this number may increase even further if epidural rates rise and if women experience prolonged labour more frequently as a result of attempts to bring down the Caesarean section rate.

Pressure sores occur when tissue is compressed between bone and the exterior surface, and depending on the situation, this may be for as little as 30 minutes.[22] Risk factors include damp skin (which is sometimes difficult to control when a woman has ruptured membranes) and steroid treatment (and in pregnancy there is a natural increase in cortisol levels).[22]

Pressure area injuries may be caused by compression, friction and/or sheer injury when a woman moves, as well as by immobility. It is all too easy to see how a woman may remain immobile for some time if, for instance, she has an epidural, a Syntocinon infusion is running, and the continuous fetal heart monitor is showing a sub-optimal trace. Both the midwife and the woman will be more concerned about not disturbing the quality of the trace by maternal movement, and much time can pass unnoticed. After delivery, a sore perineum or Caesarean section wound may restrict movement.

The Waterlow risk assessment tool[23] has been used in nursing for many years in order to identify patients at risk of developing pressure sores. However, many of its criteria are not appropriate to the childbearing population. A scoring tool for identifying risk has now been developed by a midwife and is currently being piloted.[22] This may be a valuable resource, as National Institute for Clinical Excellence (NICE) guidelines[24] recommend that risk assessment for pressure areas should include formal procedures and start within 6 hours of admission in acute episodes (e.g. labour wards). However, nothing will ever be as effective as the aware and vigilant midwife who is using her skills to ensure that the woman's condition is not compromised.

Antibiotic-resistant infection

The most well-known antibiotic-resistant infection is MRSA (methicillin-resistant *Staphylococcus aureus*). It has been known in the UK since the 1960s, and is thought to be present in most hospitals.[25] The development of resistance is believed to be directly related to inappropriate use of antibiotics (unnecessary, frequent or prolonged use, or lack of adherence to prescription instructions) and the common use of antibiotics in agriculture and aquaculture.[26]

Antibiotic-resistant bacteria are spread in the same way as any other bacteria, and can also be carried by healthcare workers who show no symptoms. MRSA often colonises the nose, and vancomycin-resistant enterococcus (VRE) can be found in the gastrointestinal tract. However, transfer is usually via contaminated hands in particular, or via contaminated equipment.

Although infection of a wound with antibiotic-resistant bacteria has been reported in the postnatal period, to date recovery has eventually been achieved. Because the infection may not be diagnosed until after the woman has left hospital, and has probably also been discharged from midwifery community care, midwives may have limited experience of these infections. However, the death of a newborn baby from MRSA was described recently in a midwifery journal, as was the devastating effect of this on the midwives,[27] and this may serve to act as a timely reminder of the dangers. Chapter 9 contains a section on handwashing, which is directly relevant to this subject.

The increase in antibiotic-resistant infection has led to initiatives to try to reduce antibiotic use. Research from France has demonstrated that antibiotic usage can be reduced in a hospital environment with the agreement of all involved.[28] This study demonstrated that from an initial audit, unjustified (according to consensual criteria) prescriptions dropped from 6% to 0%, although this figure later increased to 3%.

There is no doubt that antibiotics can be a life-saving intervention. However, it must be more appropriate to consider strengthening the immune system and good anti-infection practices as a first line of defence and treatment.

Box 8.2   Definition of sepsis[29]

Sepsis is a systemic response to infection manifested by two or more of the following:

- temperature $>38°C$ or $<36°C$
- heart rate >100 beats/minute
- respiration >20 breaths/minute or $PcCO_2$ $<32\,mmHg$
- white cell count $>17 \times 10^9$ litre or $<4 \times 10^9$ litre or 10% immature forms

plus
- bacteraemia (i.e. positive blood cultures) *or*
- positive swab culture.

Chorioamnionitis (or intra-amniotic infection)

Chorioamnionitis may be present in 1–5% of term pregnancies and up to 25% of preterm labours.[30] Most of these infections will involve organisms of the normal vaginal flora. Infected women may present with pyrexia and/or non-specific abdominal pain, but chorioamnionitis is often asymptomatic. However, it has been reported to be associated with a lack of variability[31] or fetal bradycardia[32] on cardiotocography (CTG) monitoring.

The infection can be ascending, even with intact membranes, and it has been shown that in a twin pregnancy the amniotic fluid sac closest to the os is the most usual (or only) one affected.[33] Histological chorioamnionitis increases in preterm labour or preterm pre-labour rupture of the membranes,[34] and is also associated with intrauterine growth restriction of the fetus.[35] Many otherwise unexplained stillbirths may be due to ascending infection.[36]

If the infection is undetected and untreated antenatally and in labour, the mother is at risk of developing endometritis.

Endometritis (or uterine infection)

In the UK, puerperal fever was once a frequent cause of death of newly delivered women,[37] and in areas of the world where asepsis, antibiotics and maternal good health are not common, it is still a major concern.[38]

It is difficult to determine the number of women who develop endometritis, as cultures are usually difficult (the organisms that commonly cause endometritis are frequently normal vaginal organisms). Endometritis is associated with retained products. These may be detected by ultrasound examination, but this may be inconclusive.[39] The risk factors for endometritis include previous vaginal infections, a history of preterm labours with or without rupture of membranes, prolonged rupture of membranes, prolonged labour (or labour which involved many interventions, in particular many vaginal examinations) or Caesarean section. Risk factors also include those related to the risk of wound infection (*see* Box 6.4 in Chapter 6), and of course any factor that suppresses the immune system (*see* Chapter 2).

Diagnosis is made on the basis of clinical signs (*see* Box. 8.3), and once endometritis is suspected, the tendency is to treat it swiftly, as it is known that the infection has the potential to cause serious morbidity or even death.

Box 8.3   Signs of endometritis

Pyrexia (usually >37.8°C) with no other identifiable cause
Tachycardia
Sub-involution of the uterus
Uterine tenderness
Increase or decrease in lochia
Offensive lochia
General malaise

Septic shock

Septic shock can develop either slowly or quickly, and can complicate many of the usual events or procedures that are dealt with routinely by midwives.

In a study that investigated the causes of septic shock in 18 women, pyelonephritis was the commonest cause, followed by chorioamnionitis and endometritis.[40] Amniocentesis has been reported to be one of the possible triggers for chorioamnionitis,[41] and the two most recent *Confidential Enquiries into Maternal Deaths in the UK*[37,42] each described the death of a woman following infection caused by amniocentesis.

Septic shock is more common in developing countries, but *Confidential Enquiries into Maternal Deaths*[37] reported a case in the UK of overwhelming sepsis in a woman who died shortly after admission. She was systemically unwell but not pyrexial. Using other cases as examples, *Confidential Enquiries* also suggests that new emotional and behavioural changes in late pregnancy and the early postnatal period may be due to underlying pathology, and it is important to remember that advanced sepsis can cause confusion.

In septic shock the common first signs of infection, namely pyrexia and tachycardia, can rapidly develop into hypotension, hypoxaemia, acidosis, disseminated intravascular coagulopathy and finally multiple organ failure. Hypothermia may follow the initial pyrexia, and jaundice, oliguria and pulmonary oedema may be late signs. Diarrhoea, vomiting and abdominal pain may confuse the diagnosis, but these can all be symptoms of genital tract infection.

As most cases of septic shock will require admission to an intensive care unit, the midwives' main and vitally important responsibility will be to recognise the warning signs and undertake urgent referral. It is worth quoting from *Confidential Enquiries* as a timely reminder:

> Younger women may maintain their blood pressure and conceal serious illness for a long time and appear deceptively well, alert and talking before sudden cardiovascular decompensation occurs.[37]

Necrotising fasciitis

Necrotising fasciitis is a very serious wound infection that involves widespread tissue necrosis and acute systemic toxicity, with a mortality of around 40–50%. It is not a new condition, and was mentioned by Irvine Loudon in his work *The Tragedy of Childbed Fever*[43] as probably complicating puerperal fever in the 1800s.

Necrotising fasciitis has been found complicating both perineal[44] and Caesarean section[45] wounds. In reported cases of affected women after Caesarean section, it was clear that all of them had received prophylactic antibiotics (*see* Chapter 6) and their infections were identified after hospital discharge.[45]

Because it is the underlying (hidden) tissue that is destroyed initially, careful observation needs to be made of areas of oedema and cellulitis around the wound. If these areas appear to be spreading, together with increasing pain, very rapid referral and treatment needs to be undertaken, as delays in intervention can be fatal. Pyrexia is also a common sign, along with copious and persistent discharge, dusky discoloration of the skin and/or increasing anaesthesia around the wound.

References

1 Kinlay J, O'Connell D and Kinlay S (1998) Incidence of mastitis in breastfeeding women six months after delivery: a prospective cohort study. *Med J Aust.* **169:** 310–12.

2 Fetherston C (1997) Characteristics of lactation mastitis in a Western Australian cohort. *Breastfeed Rev.* **5:** 5–11.

3 Renfrew M, Fisher C and Arms S (1990) *Breastfeeding: getting breastfeeding right for you.* Celestial Arts, Berkeley, CA.

4 Bick D, MacArthur C, Knowles H *et al.* (2002) *Postnatal Care: evidence and guidelines for management.* Churchill Livingstone, Edinburgh.

5 Wambach K (2003) Lactation mastitis: a descriptive study of the experience. *J Hum Lactation.* **19:** 24–34.

6 Fetherston C (1998) Risk factors for lactation mastitis. *J Hum Lactation.* **14:** 101–9.

7 Inch S and Renfrew M (1989) Common breastfeeding problems. In: I Chalmers, M Enkin and M Keirse (eds) *Effective Care in Pregnancy and Childbirth. Volume 2.* Oxford University Press, Oxford.

8 Cable B, Stewart M and Davis J (1997) Nipple wound care: a new approach to an old problem. *J Hum Lactation.* **13:** 313–18.

9 Buchanan P, Hands A and Jones W (1999) Cracked nipples and moist wound healing. *Breastfeeding Network.* **9:** 9–13.

10 Francis-Morrill J, Heinig J, Papagianis D *et al.* (2004) Diagnostic value of signs and symptoms of mammary candidosis among lactating women. *J Hum Lactation.* **20:** 288–95.

11 Robertson J and Herbert D (1994) Gynecologic urology. In: A DeCherney and M Pernoll (eds) *Current Obstetric and Gynaecological Diagnosis and Treatment* (8e). Prentice Hall, London.

12 D'Souza Z and D'Souza D (2004) Urinary tract infection during pregnancy – dipstick urinalysis vs. culture and sensitivity. *J Obstet Gynaecol.* **24:** 22–4.

13 Spellacy W (1996) Urinary tract infections. *Contemp Obstet Gynecol.* **41:** 23–30.

14 Smaill F (2003) *Antibiotics for Asymptomatic Bacteriuria in Pregnancy (Cochrane Review). The Cochrane Library. Issue 2.* Update Software, Oxford.

15 Polivka B, Nickel J and Wilkins J (1997) Urinary tract infection during pregnancy: a risk factor for cerebral palsy? *J Obstet Gynecol Neonatal Nurs.* **26:** 405–13.

16 Craigo S and Kapermick P (1994) Postpartum haemorrhage and the abnormal puerperium. In: A DeCherney and M Pernoll (eds) *Current Obstetric and Gynaecological Diagnosis and Treatment* (8e). Prentice Hall, London.

17 Schwartz M, Wang C, Eckhert L *et al.* (1999) Risk factors for urinary tract infection in the postpartum period. *Am J Obstet Gynecol.* **181:** 547–53.

18 Stray-Pederson B, Balkstad M and Bergan T (1990) Bacteriuria in the puerperium. *Am J Obstet Gynecol.* **162:** 792–7.

19 Jepson R, Mihaljevic L and Craig J (1999) *Cranberries for Preventing Urinary Tract Infections (Cochrane Review). The Cochrane Library. Issue 4.* Update Software, Oxford.

20 Jepson R, Mihaljevic L and Craig J (1999) *Cranberries for Treating Urinary Tract Infections (Cochrane Review). The Cochrane Library. Issue 4.* Update Software, Oxford.

21 Newton H and Butcher M (2000) Investigating the risk of pressure damage during childbirth. *Br J Nurs.* **9 (Suppl. 1):** S20–6.

22 Oliver F (2003) Pressure area care – not relevant to maternity units? *MIDIRS Midwifery Digest.* **13:** 496–7.

23 Waterlow J (1988) Prevention is cheaper than cure. *Nurs Times.* **84:** 69–70.

24 National Institute for Clinical Excellence (2001) *Pressure Ulcer Risk Assessment and Prevention.* National Institute for Clinical Excellence, London.

25 Ayliffe G *et al.* (2000) *Control of Hospital Infection: a practical handbook* (4e). Arnold, London.

26 Tenover F and Hughes J (1996) The challenge of emerging infectious diseases: development and spread of multiply resistant bacterial pathogens. *JAMA.* **275:** 300–4.

27 News (2005) Midwives devastated by MRSA baby death. *Pract Midwife.* **8:** 8.

28 Saizy-Callaert S, Causse R, Furhman C *et al.* (2003) Impact of a multidisciplinary approach to the control of antibiotic prescription in a general hospital. *J Hosp Infect.* **53:** 177–82.

29 Bewley S, Wolfe C and Waterstone M (2002) Severe maternal morbidity in the UK. In: A MacLean and J Neilson (eds) *Maternal Morbidity and Mortality.* RCOG Press, London.

30 Armer T and Duff P (1991) Intra-amniotic infection in patients with intact membranes and preterm labour. *Obstet Gynecol Surv.* **46:** 589–93.

31 De Felice C, DiLio L, Parrini S *et al.* (2004) Persistent fetal heart rate hypo-variability: a presenting clinical sign of histologic chorioamnionitis at term gestation. *J Matern Fetal Neonatal Med.* **16:** 363–5.

32 Presta G, Rosati E, Giannuzzi R *et al.* (2004) Prolonged fetal bradycardia as the presenting clinical sign in *Streptococcus agalactiae* chorioamnionitis. *J Perinat Med.* **32:** 535–7.

33 Bergstrom S (2001) Bacterial and viral infections in pregnancy: chorioamnionitis. In: J Lawson, K Harrison and S Bergstrom (eds) *Maternity Care in Developing Countries.* RCOG Press, London.

34 Sebire N, Goldin R and Regan L (2001) Histological chorioamnionitis in relation to clinical presentation at 14–40 weeks of gestation. *J Obstet Gynaecol.* **21:** 242–5.

35 Williams M, O'Brien W, Nelson R *et al.* (2000) Histological chorioamnionitis is associated with fetal growth restriction in term and preterm infants. *Am J Obstet Gynecol.* **183:** 1094–9.

36 Tolockiene E, Morsing E, Holst E *et al.* (2001) Intrauterine infection may be a major cause of stillbirth in Sweden. *Acta Obstet Gynecol.* **80:** 511–18.

37 Lewis G (ed.) (2004) *Why Mothers Die: confidential enquiries into maternal deaths in the UK 2000–2002.* RCOG Press, London.

38 Harrison K and Lawson J (2001) Puerperal disorders. In: J Lawson, K Harrison and S Bergstrom (eds) *Maternity Care in Developing Countries.* RCOG Press, London.

39 Carlan S, Scott W, Pollack R *et al.* (1997) Appearance of the uterus by ultrasound immediately after placental delivery with pathologic correlation. *J Clin Ultrasound.* **25:** 301–8.

40 Mabie W, Barton J and Sibai B (1997) Septic shock in pregnancy. *Obstet Gynecol.* **90:** 553–61.

41 Winer N, David A, Leconte P *et al.* (2001) Amniocentesis and amnioinfusion during pregnancy: report of four complicated cases. *Eur J Obstet Gynecol Reprod Biol.* **100:** 108–11.

42 Lewis G (ed.) (2001) *Why Mothers Die: confidential enquiries into maternal deaths in the UK 1997–1999.* RCOG Press, London.

43 Loudon I (2000) *The Tragedy of Childbed Fever.* Oxford University Press, Oxford.

44 Sutton (1985) Group B streptococcus necrotizing fasciitis from episiotomy. *Obstet Gynecol.* **66:** 733.

45 Goepfert A, Guinn D, Andrews W *et al.* (1997) Necrotizing fasciitis after caesarean delivery. *Obstet Gynecol.* **89:** 409–12.

9

Infection control around childbirth: the midwife's role

with the increasing tide of antibiotic resistance, basic hygienic practices may be all we have left.[1]

It has been clearly identified in many of the previous chapters that childbirth, although a normal life experience, can stress the immune system in many ways. Although the vast majority of women who receive midwifery care may not actively demonstrate the presence of a clinical infection, there is no doubt that many midwifery actions have the potential to cause an infection. If the woman's immune system then manages to cope with and overcome this invasion, then although she may not develop an infection, she is using energy and resources in the process that could be better utilised in healing, breastfeeding, coping with the demands of motherhood, and so on. Perhaps the overwhelming fatigue that most women report during the postnatal period[2] could be partially alleviated if everything possible was done to ensure that the immune system of new mothers did not have to be activated to deal with preventable pathogen loads.

Two of the areas in which midwives could perhaps make a difference are:

1 awareness of the midwife's own role in the potential spread of infection and of the ways to minimise it
2 awareness of what actions a midwife can take to protect herself.

Handwashing

In 1847, the Austrian obstetrician Ignaz Semmelweiss in Vienna was the first to identify the connection between handwashing and reducing puerperal sepsis. He demonstrated that as a result of ensuring that medical students washed their hands in chlorine water before caring for labouring women, the puerperal sepsis rate fell from 11.4% to 1.27%.[3] However, his work was initially ignored, and in this country the work of Pasteur and Lister in the 1880s, focusing on the theory of germs together with antisepsis, was fundamental in changing practice, albeit slowly.[4]

Handwashing in the early 1900s was a time-consuming and vigorous task. Hands were expected to be cleaned by:

> *a 10-minute scrub of hands with a nail brush, hot water and tincture of green soap, either with running water or at least four changes of water in a basin. Water should be boiled and filtered.*[4]

Even imagining such a regime should make current day recommendations (*see* Boxes 9.1 and 9.2) a positive pleasure! However, there is evidence that basic handwashing is a skill which is much neglected by all levels of healthcare professionals[5] – so much so that the emphasis of much of the publicity aimed at increasing handwashing is directed at the public, suggesting that they remind healthcare workers to wash their hands.

Box 9.1   Three stages of effective handwashing[6]

1 **Preparation.** Wet the hands under tepid running water before applying liquid soap or an antimicrobial preparation.
2 **Washing and rinsing.** The handwash solution must come into contact with all of the surfaces of the hands. Rub the hands together vigorously for a minimum of 10–15 seconds. Pay particular attention to the tips of the fingers, the thumbs and the areas between the fingers. Rinse the hands thoroughly.
3 **Drying.** Dry the hands with good quality paper towels.

Many of the suggested regimes are for nurses and may not be applicable to midwives on a postnatal or antenatal ward, but on a labour ward, where the midwife may put on and remove gloves and handle bed linen, clothing, etc. contaminated with liquor or blood and also handle common equipment (e.g. sphymomanometers, sonicaids) very frequently, she obviously needs to wash and disinfect her hands often. The close contact that midwives may have with women in labour (e.g. using massage or a comforting hug) may not feel like a clinical procedure, but will still need the same amount of care to prevent the spread of infection. Caring for one woman at a time will certainly reduce the opportunity for cross-infection, but this is not always possible, and even in the best of circumstances there is the scenario of a labour ward emergency where all of the available midwives will need to attend and give care.

Recently much publicity has been given to the issue of handwashing and hospital staff, and the National Patient Safety Agency (NPSA) mounted a campaign called Hand Hygiene Project[5] which, among other initiatives, sought to raise awareness among patients and visitors as well as among staff. In their initial pilot study they noted that staff cleaned their hands between patients on 76% of occasions, compared with the 28%[7] observed before the campaign. This improvement was largely achieved by making alcohol-based hand rubs easily available.

Box 9.2 Use of alcohol-based hand rub solution[6]

1 Ensure that the hands are free of dirt and organic material.
2 The hand rub solution must come into contact with all of the surfaces of the hand. Pay particular attention to the tips of the fingers, the thumbs and the areas between the fingers.
3 Ensure that the solution has evaporated and the hands are dry.

All NHS acute trusts should have alcohol-based hand rubs in place where necessary by April 2005[8] and trusts are individually responsible for auditing this practice. There is much evidence to support this strategy. For example, a study conducted in Switzerland over a period of three years throughout a teaching hospital found that supplying bedside hand rubs decreased the rate of infections from 16.9% to 9.9% and decreased cases of MRSA from 2.16 to 0.93 episodes per 10 000 patient days. The consumption of alcohol-based hand rub increased from 3.5 to 15.4 litres per 1000 patient days during this time.[9]

However, alcohol-based hand rubs are only a supplement to handwashing with cleanser and water (*see* Box 9.3 for suggestions on when hands should be washed).

Handwashing must be undertaken with the correct technique and at the right time – this is more important than the length of time or the agent used. The most commonly missed areas are the fingertips and palms,[10] and these are the areas most likely to be contaminated.

Liquid soap containers or alcohol-gel dispensers can be easily contaminated. It is important that taps and dispensers can be operated with a foot, wrist or elbow and that they are cleaned regularly.

Box 9.3   Hands should be washed:

- On arrival and when leaving the ward, the clinic or the woman's home
- When the hands are visibly dirty
- After using the toilet
- Before handling food or medicines
- Before handling a baby
- After attending to infected women or babies
- Before and after using aseptic techniques
- After handling any potentially contaminated materials or equipment (e.g. communal pens)
- After removing gloves (see information concerning gloves later in this chapter)

It is also important for the midwife to care for her hands, as such frequent cleaning can lead to dry, cracked skin which could predispose her to infection. Frequent use of handcreams may reduce this risk.

Midwifery procedures

Aseptic technique

Asepsis or aseptic technique is a method of preventing contamination by only allowing sterile fluids, instruments, etc. to come into contact with vulnerable areas. The risk of airborne contamination must also be reduced.

Aseptic technique has been practised since the early 1900s, and it is a necessary part of many midwifery practices.

Injections and intravenous procedures

Intravenous cannulation should be an aseptic procedure that involves wearing gloves, disinfecting the skin and not palpating the site after cleaning. Removal of a cannula should similarly be undertaken with due care. Peripheral cannulae should be re-sited every 48–72 hours. If any signs of infection are present, the cannula should be removed and the tip cultured.

The administration set should be changed at least every 72 hours[10] unless long-term (96 hours) filters are used.[11]

Some research[12] shows that there is no need to disinfect the skin before an injection, except for intravenous injections, although it is suggested that patients whose skin is contaminated with Gram-negative bacilli in particular are at risk. Since a woman who is giving birth on a bed may well have heavy contamination on her thighs, it may be good practice to clean the area with an alcohol swab (and let it dry) prior to administering an intramuscular oxytocic injection.

There is an added risk of infection if three-way taps are used, but the use of protective caps and cleaning with 70% alcohol before injecting will decrease this risk.[10]

Vaginal examinations

Vaginal examinations have the potential to transfer pathogens from outside the body to the upper part of the vagina, the cervix and (when the membranes are ruptured) directly to the interior of the uterus and to the fetus. It is obviously important to ensure that all vaginal examinations are necessary and are not being performed just as a routine procedure, in order to minimise this risk.

There is some evidence that the use of tap water, rather than antiseptics (which could potentially kill the normal protective commensals present), for vulval and perineal cleansing prior to vaginal examinations and normal delivery results in a reduction in infection rates.[13] If this is so, the lubricant that is used should also be non-antiseptic. However, further research on these procedures may be necessary.[14]

Urinary (Foley) catheters

Urinary catheters were introduced in the 1920s and are still in common use on labour wards today. Mostly due to the increase in the number of Caesarean sections, as well as epidurals, they are a normal part of midwifery equipment in present-day practice, both as 'in-and-out' catheters and as indwelling Foley catheters.

The association between infection and indwelling urinary catheters has been known for as long as these catheters have been used. Bacteria can enter either through the lumen of the catheter or between the catheter and the wall of the urethra.[15]

The use of a sterile container to empty catheter bags, and the use of gloves together with careful handwashing by staff, and aseptic collection of specimens via a needle and syringe, are all good practice (*see* Box 9.4).

Careful attention to aseptic technique is also necessary when using an 'in-and-out' catheter.

Indwelling catheter tubing should be anchored with tape to the woman's thigh, as traction on the tubing from a heavy collection bag, or the tubing becoming caught during movement, can cause bladder trauma and predispose to infection.

Bacteria can enter the drainage bag and tubing, especially if the bag is tipped upside down. Therefore drainage bags should always be positioned below bladder level, kept off the floor and not obstructed. Reflux of urine is associated with infection, so when transferring the woman the tube should be clamped.[16]

Box 9.4   Good practice for urinary catheter care

- Use aseptic technique during insertion
- Use lubricant during insertion
- Empty the drainage bag only when necessary
- Use aseptic technique when obtaining a urine sample
- Wear gloves when emptying the drainage bag, followed by careful handwashing by carer
- Use a sterile container to empty the drainage bag
- Position the collection bag and tubing carefully
- Anchor the catheter tubing
- Pay attention to basic hygiene for women with catheters *in situ*

Environmental factors and the spread of infection

Concern about environmental contamination is not new. In the 1958 edition of Myles' *Textbook for Midwives*, the vulval swabbing which was a routine procedure on postnatal wards was described, and it was stated that it should be carried out before or not less than 1 hour after 'bedmaking, sweeping or dusting ... because of the danger of dust as a medium of cross-infection'.[17]

It is assumed by the public and the media that one of the causes of the rise in hospital-acquired infection (in particular the 'super-bugs') is 'dirty hospitals'. Standards have been suggested for establishing a basis for assessing hospital cleaning.[1]

As the midwife is perceived to be the main carer in the maternity unit, the standard of ward cleanliness reflects on our profession. However, since the reorganisation of hospital services the individual ward midwife has had little if any direct control over cleaning services. Even if they develop a good relationship with the domestic staff (assuming that there is continuity), most midwives will appreciate that the number of domestic staff has fallen in recent years, and with the increased workload and poor pay of these staff, the midwives may feel reluctant to add to their burden. It is not unusual to see midwives undertaking cleaning duties on most wards.

However, as the general cleanliness of ward areas has been much in the news recently, the Department of Health[18] has drawn up *A Matron's Charter: an Action Plan for Cleaner Hospitals.* Since all obstetric units should have access to a 'modern matron', and they have the authority to withhold payment for cleaning, there may now be a way for midwives to directly influence the standards of cleanliness in their working environment.

It is important to be aware that potentially dangerous infection is every-where. For example, MRSA was reported to have been present on 'sterile' goods packaging for more than 38 weeks.[19] Since a surface may appear clean after being wiped with a 'dirty' cloth, and therefore there is no way to assess its cleanliness, perhaps there should be bacterial standards for clinical surfaces, as there are for the food industry,[1] together with regular testing.

There is some evidence that patients with open wounds can acquire *Staphylococcus aureus* infection from contaminated baths.[12] It is recommended that all baths should be disinfected with a non-abrasive chlorine-releasing powder before being used by a woman with an open wound,[12] which would obviously include all women on a postnatal ward. There is also a report of an outbreak of group A haemolytic streptococcus on a postnatal ward, which was traced to a contaminated bidet.[20]

Although MRSA is most commonly transmitted via person-to-person contact, it can also be airborne. One study confirmed that the level of airborne MRSA increased dramatically after bed-making activities, and remained elevated for 15 minutes.[21] These cases demonstrate the need for vigilance by the midwife in supervising domestic and other ward staff, in order to ensure that the women in her care are not put at risk.

The operating theatre can be a particularly risky environment, and this is compounded by the fact that many of these women are undergoing an operative procedure in a vulnerable state, perhaps after many hours of labour or an antepartum haemorrhage. The bacterial air counts increase with the number of individuals in theatre and with increased activity.[12] Practices such as providing extra midwifery or paediatric staff for an unexpected problem with the newborn (and these helpers entering the theatre while the Caesarean section is in progress) will increase the infection risk. However, the alternative is initial resuscitation and care of the baby outside theatre, which really is unacceptable in these days of epidurals and parents being aware of the activity. This is an area where the awareness of staff attending may be an important factor in reducing the risk of infection.

Box 9.5   Some examples of midwifery actions that may help to prevent infections post delivery

- Correct anaemia promptly (especially pre-operatively)
- Be aware of basic cleanliness and hygiene around the woman
- Use the correct operating theatre technique (*see* Chapter 6)
- Be aware of the vulnerability of maternal wounds (*see* Chapters 5 and 6)
- Optimise nutrition (give antenatal advice, no prolonged starvation pre-operatively, feed post-operatively, provide nutritious food) (*see* Chapter 4)
- Provide high-quality wound care (*see* Chapter 3)
- Be aware of the adverse effects of sleep deprivation and stress on the immune system (*see* Chapter 2) and wound healing (*see* Chapter 3)

Protection of midwives

Midwives, with their close contact with women in their care, frequent attendance in the hospital environment and routine exposure to uncontrolled body fluids, are at high risk of pathogen contamination. Awareness of this risk should mean that all midwives take every precaution to protect themselves, and that they also pay attention to maintaining their own immune systems in order to ward off potential infection. Due to the nature of their work, midwives are at particular risk of bloodborne infections, and despite routine cover for hepatitis B, there is no such protection available for hepatitis C or HIV.

Gloves

Gloves are very valuable, not only to protect the women in their care, but also to protect midwives themselves. However, it is important not to be too complacent, as even unused gloves often have defects and so allow organisms on to the hands,[10] and users are often unaware of glove puncture during use.[22] Therefore it is important that any skin breaks on the hands (or other parts of the body, as in particular when undertaking labour care, blood or liquor splashes are common) are effectively covered at all times during midwifery work.

Gloves should be worn if there is any danger of contaminating the hands, whether when handling soiled equipment or when undertaking an activity involving body fluids. As was mentioned in the section on handwashing, the hands should be cleansed both before and after wearing gloves.

Clothing

Cotton is permeable to bacteria and moisture, and therefore plastic aprons are probably most effective for protecting staff and also for preventing cross-infection when caring for several women (*Staphylococcus aureus* can be transferred via clothing). It is interesting that most midwives would not consider suturing the perineum (a relatively controlled activity) without putting on a sterile gown, but many will perform deliveries (an activity with a high level of unforeseeable outcomes) or other invasive procedures, such as rupturing of membranes or episiotomies, without wearing protective clothing.

Needlestick injuries

Good practice (*see* Box 9.6) may minimise the risk of needlestick injury. However, accidents can happen. All midwives should be aware of the availability of post-exposure prophylactic medication[23] and how and when they should access it, should the need arise.

Box 9.6   Safe use of sharps

- Gloves should be worn when taking blood, cannulating, etc.
- Do not resheath or bend needles
- Do not pass sharps from hand to hand
- Sharps containers and blood bottles should be near enough to ensure immediate disposal without the need to carry the needle
- Sharps containers should be sealed when they are three-quarters full

---

References

1 Dancer S (2004) How do we assess hospital cleaning? A proposal for microbiological standards for surface hygiene in hospitals. *J Hosp Infect.* **56:** 10–15.

2   MacArthur C, Lewis M and Knox E (1991) *Health after Childbirth.* HMSO, London.

3   Loudon I (2000) *The Tragedy of Childbed Fever.* Oxford University Press, Oxford.

4   Rhode M and Barger M (1990) Perineal care: then and now. *J Nurse Midwifery.* **35:** 220–30.

5   Cowling P (2003) Hand cleansing: stop spreading infection – start spreading the message. *Br J Infect Control.* **4:** 5.

6   Pratt R, Pellowe C, Loveday H *et al.* (2001) Preventing hospital-acquired infections. *J Hosp Infect.* **47 (Suppl. 1):** S1–82.

7   National Patient Safety Agency (2004) *Clean Your Hands Pilot Evaluation.* National Patient Safety Agency, London.

8   National Patient Safety Agency (2004) *Patient Safety Alert.* 2 September; www.npsa.nhs.uk/advice

9   Pittet D, Hugonnet S, Harbarth S *et al.* (2000) Effectiveness of a hospital-wide programme to improve compliance with hand hygiene. *Lancet.* **356:** 1307–12.

10 Ayliffe G, Fraise A, Geddes A *et al.* (2000) *Control of Hospital Infection* (4e). Arnold, London.

11 Johnson W (1994) A time and money saver. Cost comparison of IV therapy with and without Pale 96 filters. *Prof Nurse.* **10:** 94–6.

12 Ayliffe G and English M (2003) *Hospital Infection: from miasmas to MRSA.* Arnold, London.

13 Keane H and Thornton J (1998) A trial of cetremide/chlorhexidine or tap water for perineal cleaning. *Br J Midwifery.* **6:** 34–7.

14 Magill-Cuerden J and Tebby B (2002) Audit of use of tap water for vulval and perineal cleansing. *RCM Midwives J.* **5:** 64–7.

15 Falkiner F (1993) The insertion of indwelling urethral catheters – minimizing the risk of infection. *J Hosp Infect.* **25:** 79.

16 Department of Health (2001) Guidelines for preventing infections associated with insertion and maintenance of central venous catheters. *J Hosp Infect.* **47 (Suppl.):** S39–46.

17 Myles M (1958) *A Textbook for Midwives* (3e). E & S Livingstone Ltd, Edinburgh.

18 Department of Health (2004) *A Matron's Charter: an action plan for cleaner hospitals.* Department of Health, London.

19 Dietze B, Rath A, Wendt C *et al.* (2001) Survival of MRSA on sterile goods packaging. *J Hosp Infect.* **49:** 255–61.

20 Gordon G and Lochhead D (1994) An outbreak of Group A Haemolytic streptococcus puerpal sepsis spread by the communal use of bidets. *Br J Obstet Gynaecol.* **101:** 447–8.

21 Shiomori T, Miyamoto H, Makishima K *et al.* (2000) Evaluation of bedmaking-related airborne and surface methicillin-resistant *Staphylococcus aureus* contamination. *J Hosp Infect.* **50:** 30–5.

22 Smith J and Grant A (1990) The incidence of glove puncture during caesarean section. *J Obstet Gynaecol.* **10:** 317–18.

23 Boyle M (2000) Bloodborne infections – protection for midwives. *Pract Midwife.* **3:** 48–50.

Index

Page numbers in *italic* refer to boxes or figures.